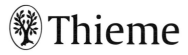
Thieme

Audiology Answers for Otolaryngologists

2nd edition

Michael Valente, PhD
Director, Division of Audiology
Department of Otolaryngology–Head and Neck Surgery
Washington University School of Medicine
Saint Louis, Missouri

Elizabeth Fernandez, AuD
Clinical Audiologist
ENT and Sleep Medicine Associates, LLC
Shiloh, Illinois

Heather Monroe, AuD
Clinical Audiologist, Dizziness and Balance Center
Department of Otolaryngology–Head and Neck Surgery
Washington University School of Medicine
Saint Louis, Missouri

L. Maureen Valente, PhD
Director of Audiology Studies
Associate Professor-Program in Audiology and Communication Sciences
Department of Otolaryngology–Head & Neck Surgery
Washington University School of Medicine
Saint Louis, Missouri

Jamie Cadieux, AuD
Supervisor, Pediatric Audiology and Cochlear Implants
Saint Louis Children's Hospital
Saint Louis, Missouri

136 illustrations

Thieme
Stuttgart • New York • Delhi • Rio de Janeiro

Foreword

I joined the Department of Otolaryngology-Head and Neck Surgery at Washington University School of Medicine in 2002 after completing a Fellowship in Head and Neck Oncology and Reconstructive Surgery. One might wonder why a Head and Neck surgeon is writing a foreword for a book about Audiology. During the years I have been a co-faculty member with Dr. Michael Valente, I have grown to know him as a dedicated and exceptional educator. Being an educator myself, these are attributes that I greatly respect. In particular, I have been impressed by his dedication to education about Audiology to health care providers both within and outside of his field. He completely understands the vital role of interdisciplinary care in today's modern world of health care delivery and the importance of education about his field to others. Most recently, we implemented a Multidisciplinary Head and Neck Cancer Clinic and Audiology has played a critical role in the design process and ultimate structure. His support and guidance for incorporating the Audiology program into this clinic structure has been nothing but spectacular.

When I learned about the 1st edition of this book several years ago, my comment to him was "Gosh, I wish I had this resource to learn from when I was a resident." This book will serve as a highly effective and efficient learning resource not only to Otolaryngologists in residencies, but I suspect also to those who are studying for board certification in Neurotology and practitioners preparing for maintenance of certification. Practitioners in many different specialties can also utilize this text as a quick Audiology clinical reference source. I know that I expect to do so. I applaud Drs. Michael Valente, Elizabeth Fernandez, Heather Monroe, Jamie Cadieux, and Maureen Valente for revising the first edition and continuing their dedication to excellence in Audiology education.

Brian Nussenbaum, MD, FACS
Vice Chair of Clinical Affairs
Division Chief, Head and Neck Surgery
Department of Otolaryngology-Head and Neck Surgery
Washington University School of Medicine
St. Louis, Missouri, USA

Foreword

Audiology has made significant advances over the last decades, now comprising a mature and robust field of broad complexity and interest. Spanning the entire lifespan, there are now a wide range of treatment options and diagnostic tests, making this growth appealing to students and seasoned professionals alike. Site of lesion testing is now commonplace and quite precise. With genetic testing, we can know if the problem is related to defects in the tectorial membrane, hair cells or spiral ganglion cells among others. New findings regarding synaptic disruption and so-called "hidden hearing loss" suggest the field will be on stable ground for many years to come. Importantly, the selection, fitting and management of implantable and non-implantable solutions have become a necessarily collaborative, multi-disciplinary activity between audiologists and otolaryngologists among others. This relationship has greatly strengthened both professions enormously.

Drs. Michael Valente, Elizabeth Fernandez, Heather Monroe, Jamie Cadieux, and Maureen Valente have created a compelling textbook for otolaryngologists so they have a greater appreciation and understanding of psychoacoustics, audiological assessment of pediatric and adult patients, amplification, vestibular assessment, and the educational training of audiologists. Students and practitioners will find *Audiology Answers for Otolaryngologists* to be engaging and instructional. Congratulations to Drs. Valente, Fernandez, Monroe, Cadieux and Valente for such a valuable contribution that will have a lasting impact for years to come.

Craig A. Buchman, MD
Lindberg Professor and Chair
Department of Otolaryngology-Head & Neck Surgery
Washington University School of Medicine
St. Louis, Missouri, USA

Preface

As in the first edition, a unique collaboration continues to exist in the Department of Otolaryngology-Head and Neck Surgery at Washington University School of Medicine, in which residents spend time observing audiologists in a variety of clinical tasks, including audiologic assessment, patient counseling, research, hearing aid fitting, and verification. This collaboration came about after the attending physicians in the Otolaryngology Department recognized that residents across the country were performing poorly on Audiology-related questions on their national board examinations. Although shadowing the day-to-day Audiology clinic is very useful to residents, not all residents will have the opportunity to experience the lifespan of patients and scope of practice in the Audiology clinic. Therefore, a supplement is necessary to ensure that residents understand all aspects of Audiology, which was the inspiration for this pocket guidebook. Because residents have incredibly demanding schedules and little extra time to wade through comprehensive Audiology textbooks to study for their board examinations, a question-and-answer format is used for this text, with concise yet detailed answers, complemented by an array of illustrations.

Audiology Answers for Otolaryngologists is divided into six chapters: Psychoacoustics, Audiometric Testing, Vestibular Evaluation, Amplification, Pediatric Audiology, and Doctoral Education in Audiology. Each chapter utilizes a question-and-answer format to provide the reader with a high-yield study guide. The answer to each question is concise yet detailed and is complemented by a figure or table to emphasize the most important information. Keywords, figure numbers, and table numbers are bolded within the text for easy reference. Chapter 1, Psychoacoustics, is the same as in the first edition and focuses on the fundamental properties related to sound and hearing. For example, this chapter provides information on sound properties such as frequency and intensity, a foundation which is necessary in order to understand audiometric interpretation and hearing aid processing. Chapters 2 and 3, Audiometric Testing and Vestibular Evaluation, respectively, are updated from the first edition. These chapters provide an indispensable guide to diagnostic Audiology that includes pure tone testing, tympanometry, and auditory brainstem response testing to videonystagmography and rotary chair testing. For Chapter 2, this edition added information on multifrequency tympanometry and ototoxic monitoring. This chapter also includes updated information on current stands. Chapter 3 in this edition was updated to include new information on vestibular evoked myogenic potentials, the video head impulse test, and the Bow and Lean test. In Chapter 4 related to Amplification, new information was added on current hearing aid technology, current standards for testing hearing aids as well an array of wireless accessories. Information was retained on patient candidacy, sound processing, hearing aid assessment, fitting, and the verification process. Chapter 5 was added to present information on evaluating the pediatric patient. Finally, Chapter 6 was added to provide the otolaryngologist with an appreciation of the educational and licensing journey audiologists undergo and provides a host of examples of how audiologists and otolaryngologists interact.

Although the primary audience of the second edition of *Audiology Answers for Otolaryngologists* continues to be ENT residents, this textbook can also be of significant use to ENT physicians, clinical audiologists, audiology students, speech-language pathologists (SLP), SLP students, and teachers of the deaf/hard-of-hearing. Because the disciplines of Otolaryngology, Audiology, Speech Pathology, and Deaf Education often work collaboratively in providing quality patient care, it is necessary to have a working knowledge of each profession. This expansion of our knowledge base outside of our own respective professions will allow us, as health care providers, to more readily understand patient reports from other disciplines, better coordinate care, and have more intellectual conversations with and about our patients. The second edition of *Audiology Answers for Otolaryngologists* is now at your fingertips. Enjoy!

1 Psychoacoustics

● What Is the Difference between dB HL and dB SPL?

The **decibel** (**dB**) is a logarithmic unit of measurement used to express the magnitude of a sound relative to some reference level. Decibels in hearing level, or **dB HL**, is commonly used in audiology because it refers to the dB level on the audiometer. The reference level for dB HL is "0," which is related to the average threshold in decibels sound pressure level (dB SPL) for the average, normal-hearing listener. In **Fig. 1.1**, the solid black line represents the average auditory threshold in dB SPL at each audiometric frequency. Each threshold in dB SPL, which is noted in the table at the bottom of **Fig. 1.1**, is equal to 0 dB HL on the audiometer for the corresponding frequency.

Decibels in sound pressure level, or **dB SPL**, refers to the magnitude of the displacement of molecules in the air. The reference for dB SPL is 20 micropascals (20 μPa) or 0.0002 dynes/cm². Because it is easy to measure dB SPL with a condenser or free-field microphone coupled to a sound level meter, sound measurements are often expressed in dB SPL.

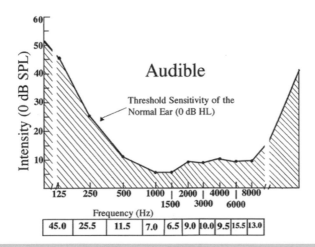

45.0	25.5	11.5	7.0	6.5	9.0	10.0	9.5	15.5	13.0

Fig. 1.1 Average thresholds across frequency in dB SPL, corresponding to 0 dB HL. For example, at 125 Hz: 0 dB HL = 45 dB SPL, and at 1,000 Hz: 0 dB HL = 7 dB SPL. (Reproduced with permission from Roeser, RJ, Clark, JL. Pure-tone tests. In: Roeser RJ, Valente M, Hosford-Dunn H, eds. Audiology: Diagnosis. 2nd ed. New York, NY: Thieme Medical Publishers, Inc.; 2007:238–260.)

● What Is the Difference between dB IL and dB SPL?

As stated in the previous section, a common method to express the magnitude of a sound is in dB SPL, for which the reference is 0.0002 dynes/cm². A less common method to express sound intensity is in acoustic power by using decibels intensity level, or **dB IL**. The reference for dB IL is 10^{-16} W/cm². According to Gulick, Gescheider, and Frisina (1989), "a dangerously intense sound would represent a power of only about 0.0024 watt" (p. 46).[1] As a result, it is cumbersome to measure the incredibly small amounts of power associated with the enormous range of intensities that the human ear can hear. Note in **Table 1.1** that the dB values are the same regardless of whether they were calculated from intensity (power) or pressure; however, a 100-fold increase in intensity is equal to a 10-fold increase in pressure.

● What Is the Difference between Detection and Discrimination?

Detection is simply the ability to determine if a sound is present or absent, whereas **discrimination** is the ability to determine the difference between two stimuli or sounds. For example, during speech audiometry patients are asked to repeat spondee words (e.g., *mushroom*, *baseball*) until a **speech recognition threshold** (**SRT**) is established. In this case, the words are increased and decreased in 5 dB steps until the audiologist finds the softest level in dB HL at which the patient can correctly repeat the word 50% of the time (hence the term speech recognition *threshold*).

Sometimes, an SRT cannot be measured and the audiologist is simply interested in measuring the level (dB HL) where the patient is aware that speech is present (**speech awareness threshold**, or **SAT**). Therefore, the SAT is a

Table 1.1 dB IL versus dB SPL

Intensity W/cm²	Times standard	dB	Dyne/cm²	Pressure times
10^{-16}	1	0	0.0002	1
10^{-14}	100	20	0.002	10
10^{-12}	10,000	40	0.02	100
10^{-10}	1,000,000	60	0.2	1,000

Source: Data from Gulick, Gescheider, and Frisina.[1]

detection measure, whereas the SRT is a threshold measure. Also, it should be clear that the dB HL associated with the SAT is lower than the dB HL associated with the SRT because one is a detection measure, whereas the other is a threshold measure.

Another common measure used by audiologists is the **word recognition score** (**WRS**). The WRS is a speech **discrimination** measure in which the patient repeats a list of 50 common, one syllable (monosyllabic) words. The words are presented at a dB level at which the listener can hear clearly, which for most normal-hearing listeners is ~40 dB louder than the listener's SRT (i.e., 40 dB SL or sensation level). The WRS is a percentage correct score (from 0 to 100%) and is useful in differential diagnosis and counseling.

● What Is the Minimum Audible Angle?

The **minimum audible angle** (**MAA**) is the smallest change in the location (azimuth) of two sound sources that can be perceived by a listener. The MAA is smallest (the listener can best identify small changes in azimuth) when the sound sources are in front of the listener (0 degrees azimuth) and is largest (poorer) when the sound sources are to the side of the listener. When sounds are directly in front of the listener, very small changes (1–2 degrees azimuth) result in an increased ability to make use of interaural differences (Gelfand, 2004)[2]; whereas when two sound sources are to the side of the listener, interaural differences remain very similar with changes in angle. **Fig. 1.2** illustrates the differences in MAA for sounds originating at 0 and 45 degrees azimuth.

● What Psychoacoustic Properties Influence Sound Localization?

One of the major advantages of binaural listening is sound localization. Differences in the arrival time and intensity of a sound between the two ears are used to determine a sound's location in space. **Interaural level difference** (**ILD**), which refers to the difference in the intensity of a sound at the two ears, is used in the localization of *high-frequency sounds* (primarily above 2,800 Hz). High-frequency sounds have wavelengths shorter than the circumference of the head and are thus influenced by the **head shadow effect**. In other words, a high-frequency sound originating to the right of a listener will decrease in intensity at the left ear due to the "roadblock"

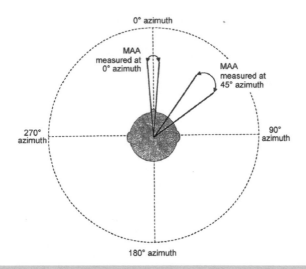

Fig. 1.2 The MAA is smallest for sounds originating directly in front of the listener, or at 0 degrees azimuth, and is largest when the sound sources are to one side of the listener. (Reproduced with permission from Gelfand.[2])

the high-frequency sound encounters at the head. In addition, spectral differences (i.e., interaural spectral differences) exist between the two ears, especially for high-frequency sounds, as spectral information is lost due to the deflection and attenuation caused by the head shadow effect. **Fig. 1.3** illustrates the difference in ILD for pure tones at various frequencies and azimuths. As can be seen from **Fig. 1.3**, the difference in intensity between the two ears at 10,000 Hz is ~20 dB when presented at 90 degrees; however, these differences lessen as the azimuth of the signal is greater than or less than 90 degrees. Also, note that as frequency decreases, the ILD decreases from 20 dB at 10,000 Hz to less than 5 dB at 250 Hz.

Interaural time difference (**ITD**) refers to the difference in the time it takes for a sound to reach each ear after the onset of a sound. Sound localization using ITDs as cues is best for *low-frequency sounds* (200–2,800 Hz). Low-frequency sounds physically have wavelengths longer than the circumference of the head; therefore, a sound originating to the right of a listener would have the same intensity and spectrum at both ears, but would arrive at the left ear later than the right ear. **Fig. 1.4** illustrates the use of ILD and ITD cues for high- and low-frequency sounds, respectively, where a sound is originating from a loudspeaker at 90 degrees azimuth or directly to the right of the listener (**Fig. 1.4a**). **Fig. 1.4b** illustrates the use of ILDs for localizing to high-frequency sounds, and **Fig. 1.4c**

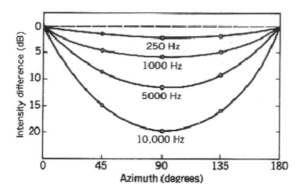

Fig. 1.3 Interaural level difference (ILD) at the ears for pure tones at 250, 1,000, 5,000, and 10,000 Hz at varying azimuths. Note that the ILD is greatest for higher-frequency tones and at 90 degrees azimuth. (Reproduced with permission from Gulick, Gescheider, and Frisina.[1])

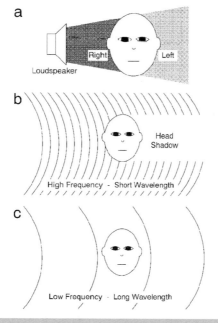

Fig. 1.4 For a sound originating at 90 degrees azimuth (**a**), interaural level differences (ILDs) assist in the localization of high-frequency sounds (**b**), and interaural time differences (ITD) assist in the localization of low-frequency sounds (**c**). (Reproduced with permission from Gelfand SA. Essentials of Audiology. 3rd ed. New York, NY: Thieme Medical Publishers, Inc.; 2009.)

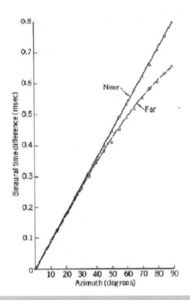

Fig. 1.5 Interaural time difference (ITD) for near and far sources at various azimuths. The ITD increases as the sound source increases from 0 to 90 degrees azimuth. (Reproduced with permission from Gulick, Gescheider, and Frisina.[1])

illustrates the use of ITDs for localizing to low-frequency sounds. At 90 degrees azimuth, the ITD is ~0.7 millisecondsec and is fairly independent of frequency. As the azimuth increases from 0 to 90 degrees, the ITD increases, as can be seen in **Fig. 1.5**.

● What Is Loudness Recruitment?

Individuals with sensorineural hearing loss may by hypersensitive to sounds that are perceived as comfortably loud to normal-hearing listeners. This "**rapid growth of loudness**" in an ear with sensorineural hearing loss is known as **recruitment** and is typically considered to be an indicator for **ochlear hearing loss** (Roeser, Valente, & Hosford-Dunn, 2007, p. 4).[3] **Fig. 1.6** illustrates one test, called loudness growth in octave bands, which had been used to measure loudness growth. As can be seen in **Fig. 1.6,** there are dashed and solid lines in each box representing loudness growth for narrowband noise centered at 500, 1,000, 2,000, and 4,000 Hz. The dashed line represents loudness growth in the normal ear at the test frequency, and the solid line represents the loudness growth at the same frequency for the listener with hearing loss. In each box, the x-axis

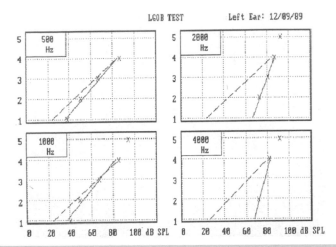

Fig. 1.6 Illustration of recruitment using the loudness growth in octave bands (LGOB) test.

represents the input signal (0–120 dB SPL), and the y-axis represents the patient's loudness judgment (on a scale of 1–5). In looking at 500 Hz, it can be seen that the patient with normal hearing goes from perceiving the signal from "very soft" (1) to "loud" (4) in a range of ~65 dB (20–85 dB SPL) and the slope of the curve is 45 degrees. At the same frequency, the hearing-impaired listener goes from soft to loud in a range of ~45 dB (40–85 dB SPL). Four things become clear. First, a loudness judgment of "1" to the hearing-impaired listener at 500 Hz required ~20 dB more input than the normal listener to obtain the same loudness judgment. This represents a 20 dB hearing loss at 500 Hz. Second, the dynamic range (DR) is ~20 dB narrower for the hearing-impaired listener. Third, the slope of the curve for the hearing-impaired listener is steeper. Fourth, the loudness judgment for the normal patient and the hearing-impaired patient is the same at the higher-input levels. Now, look at the loudness growth at 4,000 Hz. In this case, the loudness judgment for "soft" for the hearing-impaired patient is ~45 dB greater than that of the normal-hearing patient. This represents about a 45 dB hearing loss at 4,000 Hz for this patient. The DR for the normal ear is still ~65 dB wide, but for the hearing-impaired patient the DR has been reduced to ~15 dB (65–80 dB). This is recruitment! Thus, the slope of the loudness growth curve for the normal-hearing patient remains at 45 degrees, but the slope for the hearing-impaired patient is now very steep! Finally, the loudness judgment for "loud" is the same for the normal and impaired ear. Individuals with normal hearing typically have a DR, or the difference between the threshold of hearing and the level of loudness discomfort, of 100 dB SPL (**Fig. 1.7a**). Because individuals with sensorineural hearing loss have elevated thresholds and normal loudness discomfort levels (**Fig. 1.7b**), these patients have a reduced DR. As a result, small increases in intensity may be perceived as disproportionately loud to such individuals.

● What Is Frequency?

Frequency is defined as the number of cycles or repetitions per unit of time. In the International System of Units, the unit used to express frequency is hertz (**Hz**), where 1 Hz is defined as one cycle per second. The human ear has an audible frequency range of ~20 to 20,000 Hz and is most sensitive to frequencies near 1,000 Hz, as was seen in **Fig. 1.1**. The perceptual correlate of frequency is pitch, so as frequency increases a listener perceives an increase in pitch. Notice in **Fig. 1.8** that both the upper and lower waveforms represent a 1,000 Hz tone (four complete cycles in 0.004 seconds: 4/0.004 = 1,000 Hz); however, the upper waveform represents a less intense tone, as it has less amplitude than the lower waveform.

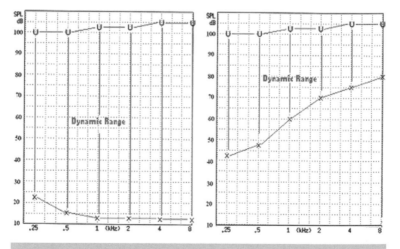

Fig. 1.7 (**a**) Dynamic range for a normal-hearing listener and (**b**) for a hearing-impaired listener plotted on an SPL-O-Gram. Unlike a traditional audiogram, which is in dB HL and goes from lowest to highest intensity (top to bottom), the SPL-O-Gram is in dB SPL and goes from highest to lowest intensity (U, uncomfortable loudness level; X, threshold).

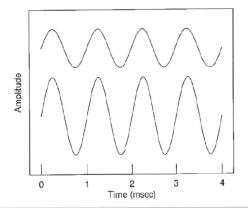

Fig. 1.8 Pure tone sinewave. (Adapted from Gelfand SA. Essentials of Audiology. 3rd ed. New York, NY: Thieme Medical Publishers, Inc.; 2009)

• What Is Fundamental Frequency and What Are Harmonics?

Fundamental frequency, abbreviated f_o, is the natural resonating frequency of a periodic signal. Harmonics are multiples of the fundamental frequency. So a fundamental frequency, f_o, would have harmonics of $2f_o$, $3f_o$, $4f_o$, etc. For example, a fundamental frequency of 1,000 Hz would have harmonics at 2,000, 3,000, 4,000 Hz, and so on. In addition, intensity decreases with each harmonic, as can be seen in **Fig. 1.9**.

• How Does the Frequency Spectrum of Vowels versus That of Consonants Influence Speech Recognition?

Vowel sounds consist primarily of low frequencies (and have more energy or are louder), whereas consonants contain more high frequencies (and have less energy or are softer). A listener's perception of "loudness" comes primarily from low-frequency sounds. On the other hand, a listener's ability to correctly discriminate two words or syllables within the same word correctly is more reliant on hearing the consonant sounds of speech. For example, it would be difficult to discriminate the difference between the words *have, has,* and *half* if the final consonants were not heard accurately. It is very common for

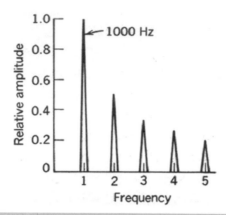

Fig. 1.9 A 1,000 Hz fundamental frequency and its harmonic frequencies, which incrementally decrease in intensity as the harmonic frequency increases. (Reproduced with permission from Gulick, Gescheider, and Frisina.[1])

individuals with presbycusis or noise-induced hearing loss, who have greater hearing loss in the high frequencies, to report that they can "hear, but not understand." These listeners have normal or near-normal low-frequency hearing (vowels), which becomes progressively poorer with increasing frequency (consonants), as shown in **Fig. 1.10**. In the audiogram in **Fig. 1.10**, sounds below the threshold line (i.e., more intense vowels) are audible, whereas sounds above the threshold line (i.e., less intense consonants) are inaudible. So it is often true that one may *hear* much of a conversation, but might *misunderstand* many words. This problem is increased in noisy environments.

● What Is the Upward Spread of Masking and How Does It Impact Speech Recognition?

Masking is simply "covering up" one sound with another. For example, if a person is talking on a cell phone while walking on a busy street, a listener may misunderstand what the person on the other line has said when a bus drives by. In this scenario, the noise from the bus is masking the telephone conversation. As the intensity of a masker increases, the masker has a greater effect on frequencies greater than the masker frequency. This phenomenon, known as the **upward spread of masking**, helps to explain why it is difficult to understand speech in the presence of background noise. Background noise, which is composed primarily of low-frequency energy,

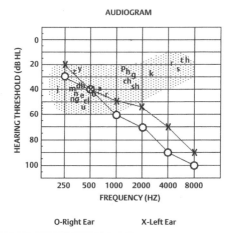

Fig. 1.10 Familiar sounds audiogram. (Reproduced with permission from Thibodeau L. Speech audiometry. In: Roeser RJ, Valente M, Hosford-Dunn H, eds. Audiology: Diagnosis. 2nd ed. New York, NY: Thieme Medical Publishers, Inc.; 2007:288–313.)

masks the higher-frequency consonant sounds of speech. As stated in the previous section, consonants contribute greatly to speech recognition abilities. So even for normal-hearing listeners, background noise can negatively impact speech recognition. This phenomenon has an even greater impact on a hearing-impaired listener, as it takes less noise to mask the high-frequency sounds and negatively impact speech recognition than for a normal-hearing listener. In addition, it is also possible for high-frequency sounds to mask lower-frequency sounds, which is known as backward masking or the **downward spread of masking**.

● What Is the Just Noticeable Difference for Intensity and Frequency?

The **just noticeable difference** (**jnd**) refers to the smallest detectable difference between two stimuli. For auditory stimuli, the jnd can be measured for intensity and frequency. The jnd for intensity varies from 0.25 to 2.5 dB and decreases as the stimulus level increases. The jnd for frequencies below 1,000 Hz is 2 to 3 Hz and for frequencies above 1,000 Hz is 0.3% of the reference frequency. For example, a listener can detect a difference between 1,000 and 1,003 Hz, but at higher frequencies (e.g., 3,000 Hz)

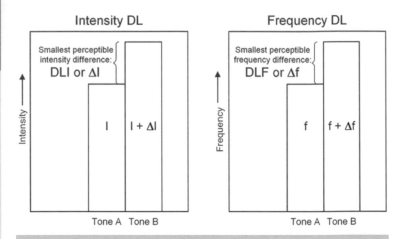

Fig. 1.11 Illustration of the just noticeable difference (jnd) for intensity and frequency. In this example, the jnd is referred to as the difference limen (DL). (Reproduced with permission from Gelfand SA. Essentials of Audiology. 3rd ed. New York, NY: Thieme Medical Publishers, Inc.; 2009.)

a greater difference (3,000 × 0.3 = 9 Hz) is required. **Fig. 1.11** provides a visual illustration of the jnd (referred to as difference limen) for intensity and frequency.

● What Are the Advantages of Binaural versus Monaural Hearing?

As stated in previous sections, input from two ears allows a listener to *localize*, or determine the location of a sound in space. Binaural hearing has additional advantages, including binaural summation and binaural squelch. **Binaural summation** refers to the perceived loudness increase when listening to a sound with both ears (of approximately equal hearing sensitivity) versus with only one ear. For example, if a listener has a threshold of 10 dB HL in both ears at 1,000 Hz, then a 1,000 Hz tone played simultaneously in both ears at 50 dB HL will sound twice as loud as the same 50 dB HL tone presented to just one ear (**Fig. 1.12**). When the intensity of a sound is near the listener's auditory threshold (0 dB SL) the binaural advantage is ~3 dB, whereas for sounds greater than or equal to 35 dB above threshold (35 dB SL), the binaural advantage is ~6 dB (Gelfand, 2004). This phenomenon is especially important in the fitting of hearing aids, as will be discussed in Chapter 4.

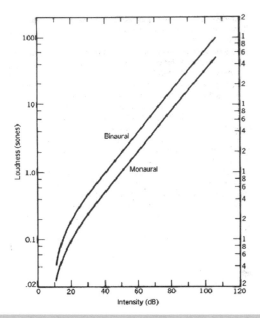

Fig. 1.12 Illustration of binaural summation. As intensity increases, perceived loudness (in sones) increases; however, the perceived loudness binaurally was twice that which was perceived monaurally. (Reproduced with permission from Gulick, Gescheider, Frisina.[1])

Binaural squelch refers to a listener's ability to listen only to the sound source of interest when additional sound sources are present. This phenomenon is commonly referred to as the **cocktail party effect**. For example, most people can recall a time at a party when several conversations were going on at once and at which time they were able to follow only the conversation of interest while tuning out all of the background noise.

When a listener has the use of only one ear or when one ear is significantly better than the other, the listener's ability to make use of localization cues is significantly reduced. In addition, monaural listening requires a greater signal-to-noise ratio (SNR = the level of the signal to the level of the noise) to communicate effectively because the advantages of binaural summation and squelch are unavailable. **Fig. 1.13** illustrates the necessary SNR improvement required for a hearing-impaired listener to perform equally as well as a normal-hearing listener in background noise. For example, if a patient has a hearing loss of 50 dB HL, he or she would have to improve the SNR by 6 dB to achieve a level

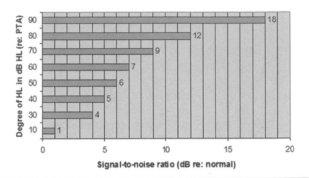

Fig. 1.13 The required signal-to-noise ratio (SNR) improvement required for a hearing-impaired listener to perform as well as a normal-hearing listener. As the degree of hearing loss increases, the SNR required to maintain performance also increases. (Reproduced with permission from Killion M. SNR loss: "I can hear what people say, but I can't understand them." *Hear Rev* 1997;4(12):8–14.)

of performance equal to that of a normal-hearing listener. Further, a patient with a hearing loss of 80 dB would have to improve the SNR by 12 dB to hear equally as well as a patient with normal hearing. There are several ways in which a hearing-impaired listener can improve his or her SNR, including the use of hearing aids with directional microphones and hearing assistance technology, such as an FM system. These devices are discussed in detail in Chapter 4.

References

1. Gulick WL, Gescheider GA, Frisina RD. Hearing: Physiological Acoustics, Neural Coding, and Psychoacoustics. New York, NY: Oxford University Press, Inc.; 1989
2. Gelfand SA. Hearing: An Introduction to Psychological and Physiological Acoustics. 4th ed. New York, NY: Marcel Dekker; 2004
3. Roeser RJ, Valente M, Hosford-Dunn H, eds. Audiology: Diagnosis. 2nd ed. New York, NY: Thieme Medical Publishers, Inc.; 2007

2 Audiometric Testing

● Why Is It Important to Calibrate Audiometric Equipment?

Audiometric equipment should be calibrated quarterly, with an exhaustive calibration required annually, to ensure that the results obtained via audiometric testing are accurate. In addition, many states require that audiometric calibration be performed annually to acquire and maintain licensure. Audiometric calibration standards are provided by the American National Standards Institute (ANSI) and by the International Electrotechnical Commission. Calibration of an audiometer involves the use of the following equipment: pistonphone (used to calibrate the sound level meter [SLM]), voltmeter, pressure and free-field condenser microphone, SLM with either an octave or one-third octave filter, appropriate couplers (6 mL, 2 mL, artificial mastoid), and a 500 g and 5.4 N (N) weight. The output of the audiometer is confirmed through the various transducers used in testing (i.e., headphones, insert earphones, bone oscillator, and loudspeaker), whereas the transducer is coupled to an artificial ear, 2-mL coupler, or artificial mastoid. For loudspeaker calibration (**Fig. 2.1d**), a calibrated free-field microphone is placed in the test room at a distance equal to where the center of a patient's head would be but with the patient absent. The output from the calibrated microphone is coupled to a calibrated SLM and one octave or one-third octave filter. Signals (narrowband noise [NBN], frequency-modulated pure tones, or speech) are sent to the loudspeaker from the audiometer, and the output from the loudspeaker is calibrated with the equipment mentioned above to be sure that the measured output adheres to the ANSI S3.6–2010 standard for sound field thresholds.[1] In ANSI S3.6–2010, there are separate standards if the loudspeaker is at 0, 45, or 90 degrees azimuth to the patient and if testing is done monaurally or binaurally. Typically, most clinics select the standard for 0 degrees with binaural hearing as their reference for sound field calibration. Reflecting back to Chapter 1 of this textbook, calibration confirms that an audiometer dial reading of 0 dB in hearing level (dB HL) is equivalent to the expected decibels in sound pressure level (dB SPL) at each frequency for all transducers. In addition, calibration verifies that no harmonic distortion exists (i.e., 1,000 Hz on the audiometer is representative of a pure tone with a frequency of 1,000 Hz), that noise interference does not exist, and that the attenuator dial is linear (i.e., an increase of 5 dB HL (on the audiometer dial) results in an increase of 5 dB SPL [in the coupler]). **Fig. 2.1** illustrates the configuration for calibration of the audiometer using the THD-49/50 headphone coupled to the 6-mL coupler (A), the ER-3A insert earphone coupled to the 2-mL coupler (B), the bone oscillator coupled to the artificial mastoid (C), and the loudspeakers being calibrated by a free-field

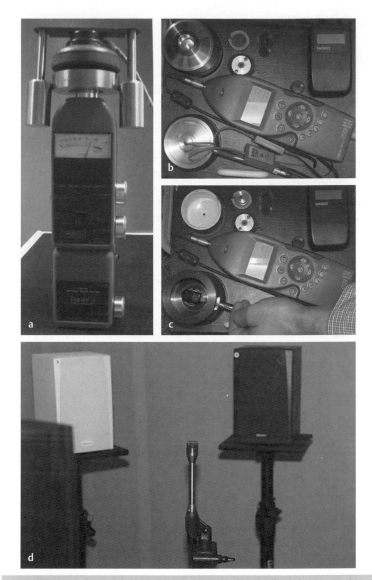

Fig. 2.1 Equipment configuration for audiometric calibration: (**a**) TDH 49/50 headphone placed on a 6-mL coupler, (**b**) ER-3A insert earphone in a 2-mL coupler, (**c**) bone oscillator on artificial mastoid, and (**d**) sound field loudspeakers being calibrated with a free-field microphone. Note: For calibration of the headphone and bone oscillator, a 500 g and 5.4 N weight, respectively, would be placed atop the transducer to simulate the appropriate tension of the headband.

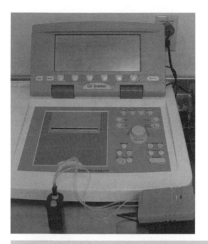
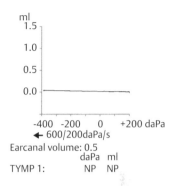

Fig. 2.2 Calibration of an immittance audiometer. (**a**) The immittance probe is placed into a 0.5-mL cavity (or a 2.0-mL cavity). A diagnostic tympanogram is performed with the probe in the coupler and (**b**) the expected result for properly calibrated equipment is displayed at right. A flat tympanogram is obtained with an ear canal volume of 0.5 mL, which is equal to the volume of the calibration cavity.

microphone (D). In addition, regular calibration should be performed on immittance audiometers to confirm that the results obtained in tympanometry, acoustic reflex threshold (ART) testing, and acoustic reflex decay testing are accurate. **Fig. 2.2** illustrates the calibration of an immittance audiometer with the use of a 0.5-mL cavity. Impedance audiometers must conform to ANSI S3.39–1987 (revised 2012) standards.[2]

● What Is the Maximum Allowable Noise Level in the Test Environment?

When measuring hearing thresholds, it is important that the noise level in the test environment does not result in erroneously elevated thresholds. According to the ANSI S3.1–1999 (revised 2013),[3] when testing pure tone thresholds using conventional (TDH-49/50) headphones the maximum permissible ambient noise levels (MPANLs) range from 16 to 33 dB SPL (**Table 2.1**, column 2) depending on test frequency. In addition, the MPANLs for testing with loudspeakers in the sound field or via bone conduction are even lower (6–16 dB SPL; **Table 2.1**, column 4), whereas those for testing using insert earphones are higher (42–51 dB SPL; **Table 2.1**, column 3). The ambient noise levels in a "quiet" office will almost always exceed the MPANLs; therefore, special care

Table 2.1 One-third octave band MPANLs (in dB SPL) for audiometric testing from 250 to 8,000 Hz

Frequency	TDH	Insert	Ears open (sound field/bone conduction)
250	20.0	48.0	16.0
500	16.0	45.0	11.0
800	19.0	44.0	10.0
1,000	21.0	42.0	8.0
1,600	25.0	43.0	9.0
2,000	29.0	44.0	9.0
3,150	33.0	46.0	8.0
4,000	32.0	45.0	6.0
6,300	32.0	48.0	8.0
8,000	32.0	51.0	9.0

Source: Data from Frank T, Rosen AD. Basic instrumentation and calibration. In: Roeser RJ, Valente M, Hosford-Dunn H, eds. Audiology: Diagnosis. 2nd ed. New York, NY: Thieme Medical Publishers, Inc; 2007:195–237.

should be taken when interpreting hearing tests obtained in rooms that do not meet ANSI S3.1–1999 (revised 2013). Further, if acceptable noise levels cannot be achieved, then the use of a single- or double-walled soundbooth is required.

● How Are Air-Conduction and Bone-Conduction Thresholds Determined?

Conventional pure tone audiometry consists of air-conduction (AC) and bone-conduction (BC) testing. AC testing involves the use of a headphone (**Fig. 2.3a**) or insert earphone (**Fig. 2.3b**) that delivers the stimulus (250, 500, 1,000, 2,000, 3,000, 4,000, 6,000, and 8,000 Hz) to the external auditory canal. The thresholds obtained via AC testing reflect the status of the outer ear, middle ear, and inner ear. BC testing involves the use of a bone oscillator (**Fig. 2.3c**) to deliver the stimulus (250, 500, 1,000, 2,000, 3,000, and 4,000 Hz) to the mastoid process. The thresholds obtained via BC testing reflect the status of only the inner ear. Thresholds are typically obtained using a bracketing technique in which the audiologist increases and decreases the attenuator dial on the audiometer (dB HL) until threshold is determined. Threshold is defined as the lowest intensity level (dB HL) at which the patient hears the stimulus 50% of the time. (Note: Pure tone testing at inter-octaves of 750 and 1,500 Hz is required if a difference of 20 dB HL exists between 500 and 1,000 Hz or 1,000 and 2,000 Hz, respectively.)

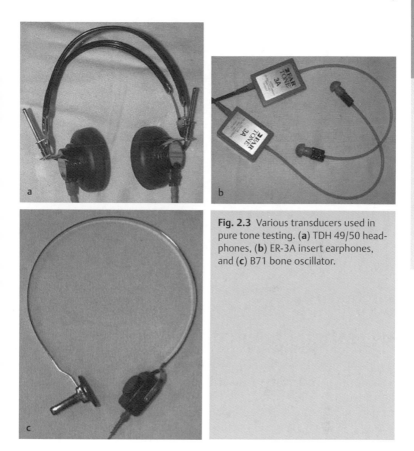

Fig. 2.3 Various transducers used in pure tone testing. (**a**) TDH 49/50 headphones, (**b**) ER-3A insert earphones, and (**c**) B71 bone oscillator.

Pure tone thresholds are plotted on an audiogram, with frequency on the x-axis and dB HL on the y-axis, using the audiometric symbols illustrated in **Fig. 2.4**. The audiogram must maintain an aspect ratio of 20 dB per octave, meaning that if the distance between 0 and 20 dB HL is 1 in, then the distance between each octave (e.g., 250–500 Hz) must also be 1 in. Pure tone thresholds for the right ear are commonly recorded using red symbols and are represented by a circle (unmasked) or triangle (masked) for AC and a bracket (with the opening facing rightward) for BC testing. Pure tone thresholds for the left ear are commonly recorded using black or blue symbols and are represented by an "x" (unmasked) or square (masked) for AC and a bracket (with the opening facing leftward) for BC testing. In some cases, a patient may have no response to pure tones at the limits of the audiometer. Such responses are recorded using the appropriate symbol (unmasked or masked AC or BC) with the addition of an arrow that points diagonally to the bottom left corner of the audiogram for right ear responses and diagonally to the bottom right corner of the audiogram for left ear responses.

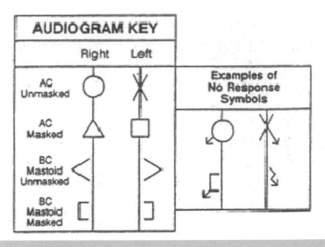

Fig. 2.4 Audiometric symbols.

● When Is Masking for Air-Conduction Testing Required?

Masking is the use of a noise source placed into the non-test ear (NTE) to prevent the participation of the NTE in the determination of a patient's audiometric threshold in the test ear (TE). The noise source used in masking for pure tone testing is NBN centered at the test frequency (e.g., 1,000 Hz NBN to NTE when establishing a threshold for 1,000 Hz in the TE). Masking for speech audiometry is conducted using a speech noise, which is a broadband noise (centered around 500–2,000 Hz) filtered to mirror the long-term average speech spectrum.

Masking for AC testing is required if the AC threshold at a test frequency in the TE exceeds the BC threshold of the NTE by 40 dB HL or greater at the same test frequency. Thus, this rule requires a contralateral comparison between the AC threshold of the TE to the BC threshold at the same frequency in the opposite or NTE. The criterion of 40 dB HL was chosen as a conservative estimate of the minimum interaural attenuation for AC testing. Interaural attenuation is the amount by which a signal introduced to the TE is decreased during transmission through the skull to the NTE.[4] **Fig. 2.5a** illustrates the crossover that occurs to the NTE when a signal of greater than or equal to 40 dB HL is introduced to the TE. The masking stimulus for all pure tone testing consists of NBN centered around the test frequency to the NTE (**Fig. 2.5b**).

● When Is Masking for Bone-Conduction Testing Required?

Masking for BC testing is required if the AC threshold of the TE exceeds the BC threshold of the TE by 10 dB HL or more, which is referred to as an air–bone gap. The minimum interaural attenuation for BC testing is 0 dB and therefore, the criterion for masking is reduced compared with that of masking for AC testing (**Fig. 2.5c**). Thus, this rule requires an ipsilateral comparison between the AC and BC threshold of the same ear at the test frequency; however, masking for BC testing is performed via an NBN centered around the test frequency to the NTE using AC. As can be seen in **Fig. 2.6**, when masking for right BC thresholds, the right ear remains unoccluded while the left ear is covered with the headphone for presentation of the masking noise. In this case, the right earphone is simply placed on the right side of the head so as not to occlude the right ear and to support the earphone placed over the left ear.

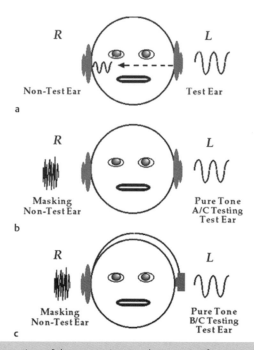

R   L

Non-Test Ear   Test Ear

a

R   L

Masking   Pure Tone
Non-Test Ear   A/C Testing
                                    Test Ear

b

R   L

Masking   Pure Tone
Non-Test Ear   B/C Testing
                                    Test Ear

c

Fig. 2.5 Illustrations of the average interaural attenuation for air-conduction testing (**a**), and masking configurations for air-conduction (**b**) and bone-conduction (**c**) testing. (Adapted from Roeser and Clark.[4])

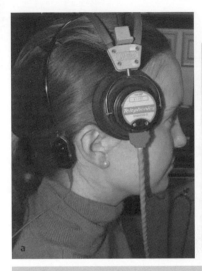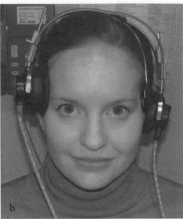

Fig. 2.6 (a,b) Transducer configuration for masked bone-conduction testing on the right ear, with masking noise presented to the left ear via the left earphone. In this case, the right earphone is simply resting on the side of the head.

● How Is the Speech Recognition Threshold Determined?

During speech audiometry, patients are asked to repeat a standardized list of spondee words (e.g., mushroom, baseball) until a speech recognition threshold (SRT) is established. In this case, the words are decreased in 10 dB steps and increased in 5 dB steps until the audiologist finds the softest level in dB HL at which the patient can correctly repeat the word 50% of the time (hence the term speech recognition threshold). The spondee words used to establish the SRT are presented via a recorded list or the audiologist may use a microphone to present the words via monitored live voice (MLV). Although recorded presentation is preferred so that results may be more reliably compared between audiologists and clinics, MLV is often used. In such cases in which MLV is used, it is important that the audiologist present each syllable of the spondee word at 0 dB on the volume units (VU) meter of the audiometer for greater accuracy. The SRT should be in good agreement (± 10 dB) with the patient's pure tone average (PTA), or the average of pure tone thresholds at 500, 1,000, and 2,000 Hz, in a reliable test session.

Sometimes, an SRT cannot be measured and the audiologist is simply interested in measuring the level (dB HL) at which the patient is aware that speech is present (speech awareness threshold, or SAT). The SAT should be

Table 2.2 Interpretation of speech recognition threshold (SRT)

SRT (dB HL)	Interpretation
0–15	Normal
16–25	Slight
26–40	Mild
41–55	Moderate
56–70	Moderately severe
71–90	Severe
> 90	Profound

in good agreement with the patient's best pure tone threshold because the SAT is merely a detection measure and does not require identification of the spondee word. **Table 2.2** summarizes the interpretation of the SRT.

● How Is the Word Recognition Score Determined?

Another common measure made by audiologists is the word recognition score (WRS). The WRS is a measure in which the patient repeats a list of 50 one-syllable (monosyllabic), phonetically balanced words, and in which a percentage correct score is calculated. For adult patients, the most common word lists are the NU-6 (male or female talker) or the CID-22 (male talker). For children, the most commonly used word list is the PBK-50. The best practice is to use a complete 50-word list unless the patient misses two or less of the first 25 words. If more than two words of the first 25 are missed, then the best practice is to administer all 50 words. Also, many audiologists unfortunately use MLV presentation of the monosyllabic words. In this practice, the audiologist uses a microphone to present the words live as he/she monitors the vocal effort (input level) of his/her presentation by observing the VU meter on the audiometer. The goal is to peak the words of the carrier phase "say the word" at 0 dB on the VU meter, but let the presentation level of the actual word fall to a more natural presentation. As one can imagine, this is not the preferred best practice as this will create significant inter- and intra-audiologist variability. Best practice demands that the 50 words be presented in a standardized format using ether a compact disc or tape presentation of the word lists. The words are presented at a dB level at which the listener can hear clearly, which for most normal-hearing listeners is ~40 dB louder than the listener's SRT (i.e., 40 dB SL, or sensation level). **Table 2.3** provides guidelines for interpreting the WRS.

Table 2.3 Interpretation of word recognition score (WRS)

WRS (%)	Interpretation
90–100	Normal
76–88	Slight difficulty
60–74	Moderate difficulty
50–58	Poor
< 50	Very poor

● When Is Masking for Speech Recognition Threshold Required?

Masking for SRT testing is required if the SRT in the TE exceeds the best BC threshold of the NTE at any of the speech frequencies (500, 1,000, or 2,000 Hz) by 40 dB or more. Masking for speech audiometry utilizes a speech noise that is presented to the NTE via AC.

● When Is Masking for Word Recognition Testing Required?

Masking for WRS testing is required when the presentation level of the words in the TE exceeds the best BC threshold of the NTE by 40 dB or more at any of the speech frequencies (500–2,000 Hz). Because word recognition testing is typically conducted at 40 dB SL (in reference to the listener's SRT in the same ear), it may be assumed that masking for WRS should always be used in patients with relatively symmetrical hearing sensitivity. Again, masking for speech audiometry utilizes a speech noise that is presented to the NTE via AC.

● How Do You Interpret an Audiogram?

Audiometric interpretation involves determining the type, magnitude, and configuration of hearing loss. As stated previously, the type of hearing loss is determined by comparing AC and BC thresholds, and may be classified as conductive, sensorineural, or mixed. The magnitude of hearing loss is interpreted on a range from normal to profound and is based on the PTA (PTA = average of thresholds at 500, 1,000, and 2,000 Hz). **Table 2.4** reports the magnitude of hearing loss.

The configuration or shape of the hearing loss can be classified as flat, sloping, rising, precipitous, trough, inverted trough, high frequency, fragmentary (corner), or notched. A flat configuration is characterized by little or no change in thresholds across frequencies (±20 dB). A sloping configuration is characterized by hearing thresholds decreasing (poorer) as frequency increases. This sloping configuration can be gradual, sharp, or precipitous. A rising configuration is characterized by hearing thresholds increasing (improving) as frequency increases. This rising configuration can be gradual, sharp, or precipitous. A precipitous configuration is characterized by hearing thresholds decreasing (poorer) very sharply between octave frequencies. A trough configuration is characterized by hearing thresholds being poorer in the mid frequencies and better in the low and high frequencies. This configuration is often associated with genetic hearing loss. An inverted trough configuration is characterized by hearing thresholds being better in the mid frequencies and poorer in the low and high frequencies. A high-frequency configuration is characterized by hearing thresholds being within normal limits at 250 to 2,000 Hz and followed by hearing loss at 3,000 to 8,000 Hz. A fragmentary (corner) configuration is characterized by hearing thresholds being present only in the very low frequencies. A notched configuration is characterized by normal hearing through 3,000 Hz with a sharp drop at 4,000 and 6,000 Hz, and improvement at 8,000 Hz. This configuration is typically seen in patients having a history of excessive exposure of loud levels of noise. Another example of a notched configuration is during BC testing when there is poorer hearing at 2,000 Hz with better hearing at 1,000 and 4,000 Hz. This is sometimes called Carhart's notch and is sometimes seen in patients with otosclerosis. **Fig. 2.7** provides illustrations and descriptions for the audiometric configurations discussed above.

Table 2.4 Interpretation of magnitude of hearing loss based upon the pure tone average (PTA), which is the average of thresholds at 500, 1,000, and 2,000 Hz

PTA (dB HL)	Magnitude of hearing loss
0–15	Normal
16–25	Slight
26–40	Mild
41–55	Moderate
56–70	Moderately severe
71–90	Severe
> 90	Profound

Term	Description	Audiometric Configuration
Flat	There is little or no change in thresholds (+ or − 20 dB) across frequencies	
Sloping	As frequency increases, the degree of hearing loss increases	
Rising	As frequency increases, the degree of hearing loss decreases	
Precipitous	There is a very sharp increase in the hearing loss between octaves	
Scoop or trough shape	The greatest hearing loss is present in the midfrequencies, and hearing sensitivity is better in the low and high frequencies	
Inverted scoop or trough shape	The greatest hearing loss is in the low and high frequencies, and hearing sensitivity is better in the midfrequencies	
High frequency	The hearing loss is limited to the frequencies above the speech range (2000–3000 Hz)	
Fragmentary	Thresholds are recorded only for low frequencies, and they are in the severe-to-profound range	
4000 to 6000 Hz notch	Hearing is within normal limits through 3000 Hz, and there is a sharp drop in the 4000 to 6000 Hz range, with improved thresholds at 8000 Hz	

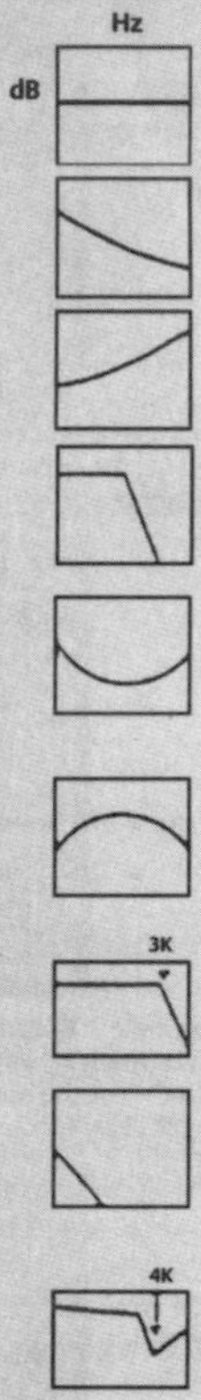

Fig. 2.7 Audiometric configuration. (Reproduced with permission from Roeser RJ, Buckley KA, Stickney GS. Pure tone tests. In: Roeser RJ, Valente M, Hosford-Dunn H, eds. Audiology: Diagnosis. 2nd ed. New York, NY: Thieme Medical Publishers, Inc; 2007:227–251.)

● What Is the Difference between Conductive, Sensorineural, and Mixed Hearing Loss?

A conductive hearing loss (CHL) is the result of an inefficient transmission of sound from the outer ear and/or middle ear to the inner ear. Foreign bodies in the ear canal, cerumen impaction, and conditions such as atresia, otitis media, and otosclerosis can result in a CHL. CHL can oftentimes be corrected medically or surgically.

A sensorineural hearing loss (SNHL) is the result of damage to the inner ear and/or the auditory nerve. Noise-induced hearing loss, presbycusis, and Meniere's disease are examples of SNHL. An SNHL is typically permanent and typically cannot be corrected medically or surgically; however, some causes of SNHL such as Meniere's disease and sudden SNHL may be improved with medical treatment.

A mixed hearing loss has both conductive and sensorineural components. For example, an individual with presbycusis and chronic otitis media with effusion may present with a mixed hearing loss.

The type of hearing loss is determined by the relationship between AC and BC thresholds. In AC testing, the stimulus is delivered via headphones or insert earphones. BC testing delivers the stimulus via vibration produced by a bone oscillator placed on the mastoid process; therefore, the signal bypasses the outer ear and middle ear and directly stimulates the inner ear. Individuals with a CHL have normal BC thresholds ($\leq$ 15 dB HL) and reduced AC thresholds. On the audiogram, this is defined by an air–bone gap greater than 10 dB or as is illustrated for the right ear ([and $\triangle$) in **Fig. 2.8a**. Patients with SNHL have AC and BC thresholds that are equally depressed, are greater than 15 dB HL, and where no air–bone gaps are present. This is illustrated in **Fig. 2.8b**, where the BC thresholds from 2,000 to 4,000 Hz are beyond the limits of the audiometer. Finally, a patient with a mixed hearing loss has decreased AC and BC thresholds with a concurrent air–bone gap (i.e., BC threshold is > 15 dB HL and there is a significant air–bone gap) as can be seen for the left ear (] and □) in **Fig. 2.8c**.

● What Are Audiometric Criteria for an Acoustic Neuroma?

Several audiometric "red flags" may be indicative of a possible acoustic neuroma.

Factors such as asymmetrical hearing loss in the high frequencies (at two or more adjacent frequencies), poor WRSs, elevated and/or absent ARTs, and positive acoustic reflex decay may be suggestive of a retrocochlear (i.e., past the cochlea) pathology. In addition to audiometric findings, subjective patient complaints of unilateral symptoms (i.e., tinnitus, aural fullness, facial numbness) should also be considered as possible indicators for

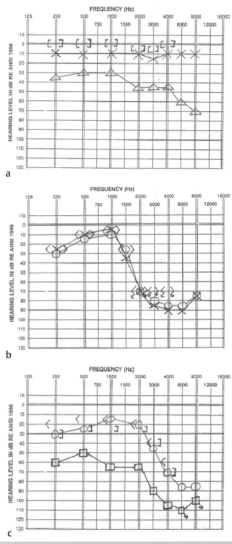

Fig. 2.8 Example audiograms: conductive, sensorineural, and mixed (**a–c**). (**a**) Normal left; conductive right (mild from 250 to 1,000 Hz gradually sloping to moderately severe from 2,000 to 8,000 Hz). (**b**) Bilateral SNHL (mild rising to normal from 250 to 1,000 Hz, precipitously sloping from mild to severe from 1,000 to 2,000 Hz, with a severe trough configuration from 2,000 to 8,000 Hz). (**c**) Mild rising to slight SNHL in the right ear from 250 to 1,000 Hz that precipitously slopes to severe through 8,000 Hz; moderately severe mixed hearing loss from 250 to 2,000 Hz steeply sloping to profound mixed hearing loss from 4,000 to 8,000 Hz in the left ear.

retrocochlear pathology, especially on the side with the expressed symptoms. When one or more of the aforementioned red flags are present, it is always recommended that the patient follow up with an otologist to rule out a retrocochlear pathology, which often involves auditory brainstem response (ABR) testing and medical imaging.

● What Is Tympanometry and How Is It Interpreted?

Tympanometry is an objective measure of middle ear function, which determines the amount of energy transmitted by the middle ear system. This measurement is obtained by placing a probe in the ear canal that consists of three ports: a loudspeaker, manometer pressure pump, and microphone. **Fig. 2.9** shows an immittance audiometer with the probe indicated by the solid arrow. During tympanometry, a 226 Hz tone is introduced by the loudspeaker via the probe assembly while the manometer pressure pump automatically and slowly varies the pressure in the ear canal from +200 to –200 daPa (dekapascals). In the meantime, the microphone in the probe assembly measures the change in intensity (in dB SPL) as the pressure is varied. As immittance decreases (i.e., the eardrum is stiffer and more sound is reflected off the tympanic membrane), the measured SPL increases. As immittance increases (i.e., the eardrum is more compliant

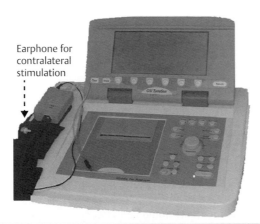

Earphone for contralateral stimulation

Fig. 2.9 Example of an immittance audiometer used to perform tympanometry, acoustic reflex thresholds, reflex decay, and eustachian tube function testing. The probe assembly is indicated by the solid arrow and the insert for contralateral stimulation by the dashed arrow.

Table 2.5 Interpretation of tympanometry

Parameter	Normal range
Ear canal volume	0.6–1.5 mL
Middle ear pressure	± 100 daPa
Static admittance	0.3–1.4 mmhos

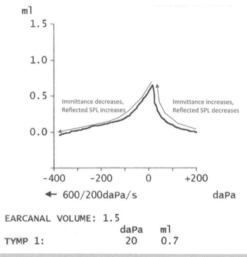

Fig. 2.10 Example of a normal tympanogram.

and less sound is reflected off the tympanic membrane), the measured SPL decreases. When completing tympanometry, the audiologist is measuring ear canal volume (ECV) (physical space between the end of the probe assembly and the tympanic membrane), middle ear pressure (MEP) (i.e., pressure along the abscissa of the tympanogram where the eardrum is the most compliant or where pressure is equal on both sides of the tympanic membrane), and static admittance or maximum compliance (point along the tympanogram where the amount of reflected SPL is the least).

In the normal adult middle ear, the ECV would be between 0.6 and 1.5 mL, the MEP would be ±100 daPa, and the maximum compliance (i.e., height of the tympanogram) would be between 0.3 and 1.4 mL. **Table 2.5** provides normative values for the interpretation of tympanometry, and **Fig. 2.10** illustrates a normal tympanogram. If the ECV is 1.5 mL, then this may suggest the presence of a perforation of the tympanic membrane or a functioning pressure equalization tube (**Fig. 2.11a**, where ECV is 7.2 mL). An ECV of less than 0.60 mL may suggest a cerumen plug, blocked probe

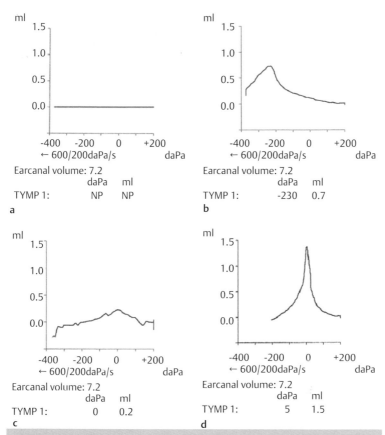

Fig. 2.11 Abnormal tympanograms: (**a**) flat tympanogram accompanied by an enlarged ear canal volume (7.2 mL) consistent with a perforation or a patent tympanostomy tube, (**b**) significant negative pressure (−230 daPa), (**c**) hypocompliant tympanogram (0.2 mL), and (**d**) hypercompliant tympanogram (1.5 mL).

assembly, or an unusually small ear canal. If the MEP is greater than −100 daPa, then this might suggest the presence of a malfunctioning eustachian tube (**Fig. 2.11b**, where MEP is −230 daPa). An MEP of greater than +100 daPa may suggest the presence of acute otitis media. If the static compliance is less than 0.30 mmhos, this would suggest a "stiff" or hypocompliant middle ear system that could be related to, for example, the presence of otitis media or otosclerosis (**Fig. 2.11c**, where static compliance is 0.2 mL). If the static compliance is greater than 1.4 mmhos, this would suggest a hypercompliant middle ear system that could be related to, for example, a scarred tympanic membrane or ossicular discontinuity (**Fig. 2.11d**, where static compliance is 1.5 mL).

● What Is High Frequency Tympanometry and When Is It Indicated?

As stated previously, conventional tympanometry utilizes a 226 Hz probe tone; however, in children under 6 months of age, 226 Hz tympanometry may not yield accurate results due to incomplete ossification in the infant's ear canal. The hypercompliant ear canal in infants easily absorbs the low frequency stimulus in 226 Hz tympanometry, which may yield a normal tympanogram via 226 Hz tympanometry, even in the presence of middle ear effusion.[5,6] Tympanometry that uses a 1,000 Hz tone has been shown to more accurately assess the middle ear status of infants, as this frequency is not easily absorbed by the ear canal. The graphical representation, interpretation, and classification of 1,000 Hz tympanometry is the same as 226 Hz tympanometry.

● What Is Wideband Tympanometry and How Is It Interpreted?

In wideband tympanometry (WBT), the acoustic stimulus is a click that includes frequencies from 226 to 8,000 Hz instead of the single 226 Hz or 1,000 Hz tone that is utilized in conventional, single-frequency tympanometry. Just as we assess hearing sensitivity by obtaining pure tone thresholds that span the frequency range of human speech, it is clinically useful to obtain a wideband assessment of middle ear function. The result of WBT is a three-dimensional "mountain" consisting of hundreds of tympanograms at different frequencies and across the pressure range. A selected frequency range of tympanograms is averaged together to form the wideband tympanogram (375–2,000 Hz for adults; 800–2,000 Hz in children under 6 months of age). The wideband tympanogram looks much like a conventional tympanogram, with pressure in daPa on the x-axis; however, unlike conventional tympanometry, where static compliance in mL is plotted on the y-axis, WBT illustrates the amount of energy absorbed by the middle ear system in percentage absorbance.[5,6] **Fig. 2.12** illustrates the 3D mountain of tympanograms on the left and the averaged, wideband tympanogram on the right. The interpretation and classification of WBT is the same as conventional tympanometry with the exception that, instead of analyzing static compliance, we are analyzing percentage absorbance, with normal peak absorbance occurring between 40 and 60%.

Another way to analyze the large amount of data collected in WBT is to analyze absorbance across the frequency range. WBT results in specific

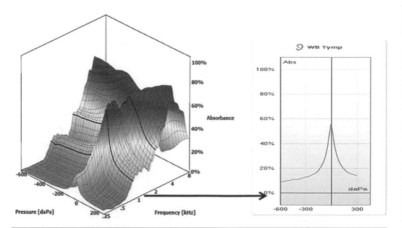

Fig 2.12 Wideband tympanometry: on the left is the 3D mountain of tympanograms and the averaged, wideband tympanogram is on the right. In this example, the wideband tympanogram is an average of frequencies from 800 to 2,000 Hz (note the solid black lines on the 3D graph).[6]

absorbance profiles for different middle ear conditions, which allows for more accurate differential diagnosis. For example, a patient with ossicular discontinuity will have a peak in absorbance in the low/mid frequencies re: the suggested normative range, whereas a patient with otosclerosis will have a reduction in absorbance in the low/mid frequencies. Wideband absorbance can be measured and/or analyzed either at tympanometric peak pressure or at ambient pressure, which is useful for patients who have a patent pressure equalization tube or tympanic membrane perforation. In addition, WBT has been found to be a better predictor of CHL when compared with traditional tympanometry.[6,7] WBT is a new test and research is still emerging on its applications; however, benefits may include better detection/monitoring of otosclerosis and ossicular discontinuity, improved detection of middle ear conditions in infants, and pre- and postoperative monitoring of conditions such as otosclerosis. **Fig. 2.13** illustrates the normative range for interpretation of wideband absorbance that is measured with a traditional pressure sweep (dynamic) or at ambient pressure (static).[8]

● What Is Eustachian Tube Function Testing and How Is It Interpreted?

Occasionally, a normal tympanogram may be recorded in patients who complain of middle ear symptoms, such as otalgia or ear pressure.

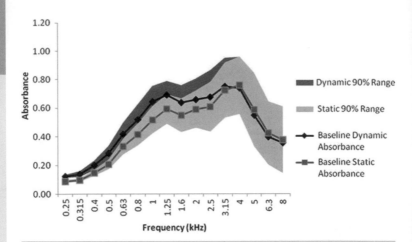

Fig 2.13 Normative range for interpretation of wideband absorbance that is measured with a traditional pressure sweep (dynamic) or at ambient pressure (static).[8]

It is important to keep in mind that a normal tympanogram does not necessarily mean normal middle ear function. In these cases, eustachian tube function (ETF) testing provides additional information regarding the middle ear status, specifically the eustachian tube's ability to open and close with auto-insufflation and after swallowing, respectively. Standard ETF testing requires the tester record three consecutive 226 Hz tympanograms: the first under normal conditions with the patient at rest, the second after the patient performs the Valsalva maneuver, and the third after the patient swallows. The peak MEP is compared between each consecutive test, and a normal ETF test yields a peak pressure shift of ≥ +10 daPa when comparing tympanogram 1 to tympanogram 2 and a ≥ −10 daPa shift when comparing tympanogram 2 to tympanogram 3. If the peak MEP shift is less than 10 daPa from one test condition to the next, then the ETF test is positive for eustachian tube dysfunction. **Fig. 2.14** illustrates a normal ETF test (A) and an abnormal ETF test (B).

● What Are Acoustic Reflex Thresholds and How Are They Interpreted?

The introduction of a loud sound to the ear canal of either ear results in the acoustic reflex, or the contraction of the stapedius muscle (and to a lesser degree, the tensor tympani) causing the tympanic membrane to stiffen and causing a resulting change in middle ear immittance. This change in

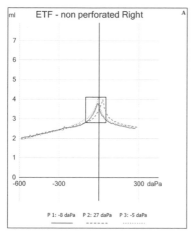
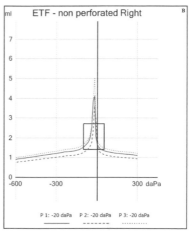

Fig. 2.14 Eustachian tube function test: a normal ETF test (**a**) and an abnormal ETF test (**b**).

immittance is measured as an increase in dB SPL by the microphone in the probe assembly. Acoustic reflex thresholds (ARTs), or the lowest level at which the acoustic reflex can be elicited (deflection = 0.02 mL), are clinically useful in the direct evaluation of middle ear status and the indirect evaluation of cochlear and retrocochlear status. ARTs can be measured ipsilaterally (stimulus is in the probe ear) or contralaterally (stimulus is in the nonprobe ear) via a supra-aural or insert earphone (indicated by the dashed arrow in **Fig. 2.9**), and are commonly measured at 500, 1,000, 2,000, and 4,000 Hz. **Fig. 2.15** illustrates the acoustic reflex pathway for ipsilateral (solid line) and contralateral (dashed line) stimulation. As can be seen in **Fig. 2.15**, the measurement of ARTs not only provides information regarding the status of the middle ear system, but also of the inner ear, auditory nerve, regions of the lower auditory brainstem, and the facial nerve.

Fig. 2.16 illustrates the tracings obtained in ipsilateral ART testing at 500 Hz (upper) and 1,000 Hz (lower). In **Fig. 2.16**, the ART at 500 Hz is 85 dB HL and at 1,000 Hz it is 80 dB HL, as this is the lowest level at which a deflection of ≥ 0.02 mL is noted (notice how below threshold the reflex amplitude is less than 0.02 and above threshold the reflex amplitude increases). ARTs are typically present between 70 and 100 dB HL in normal-hearing patients. Contralateral reflexes are generally 5 to 10 dB SL re: the ipsilateral ART at the corresponding frequency. ARTs may be present at normal sensation levels, elevated SLs, reduced SLs, or may be completely absent. **Table 2.6** summarizes the interpretation of ARTs.

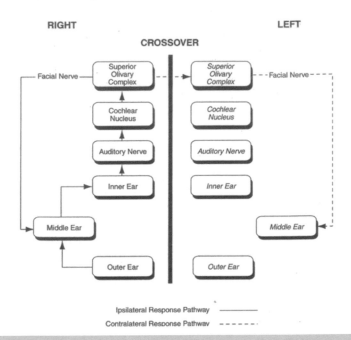

Fig. 2.15 Acoustic reflex arc illustrating right ipsilateral (solid line) and right contralateral (dashed line) pathways. (Reproduced with permission from Martin FN, Clark JG. Introduction to Audiology. Fig. 6.6. Upper Saddle River, NJ: Pearson Education, Inc.; 2006:160.)

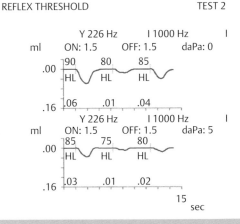

Fig. 2.16 Ipsilateral acoustic reflex thresholds (ARTs) at 500 (upper curve) and 1,000 (lower curve) Hz from a patient with normal hearing. The ART at 500 Hz was established at 85 dB HL and at 1,000 Hz was established at 80 dB HL.

Table 2.6 Interpretation of acoustic reflex thresholds

Hearing status	Expected acoustic reflex threshold (dB HL)
Normal	70–100 dB HL
Conductive loss	Elevated or absent
Cochlear loss	Normal sensation level (SL) or reduced SL
Neural loss	Normal SL, elevated, or absent

● What Is Acoustic Reflex Decay and How Is It Interpreted?

Acoustic reflex decay is a measure of the sustainability of the acoustic reflex, or how long the stapedius muscle can remain contracted during continuous stimulation. Reflex decay is measured with contralateral stimulation at 500 and 1,000 Hz at 10 dB SL (re: contralateral ART). The tone is presented continuously for 10 seconds and the patient is instructed to remain as still as possible. Negative reflex decay indicates that the magnitude of the stapedial reflex contraction did not decrease by ≥ 50% in the first 5 seconds of testing (**Fig. 2.17a**), whereas positive reflex decay indicates that the magnitude of the stapedial reflex contraction decreased by ≥ 50% in the first 5 seconds of testing (**Fig. 2.17b**). Positive acoustic reflex

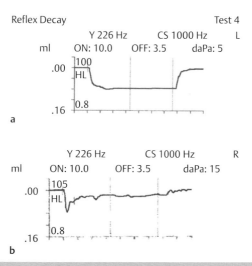

Fig. 2.17 Negative (**a**) and positive (**b**) acoustic reflex decay at 1,000 Hz.

decay may be suggestive of retrocochlear pathology and further evaluation by an otologist is strongly recommended.

● What Is the Stenger Test and How Is It Performed for Pure Tone and Speech Testing?

The Stenger test is useful in the differential diagnosis of functional hearing loss or malingering when an individual presents with an asymmetrical or unilateral hearing loss (20 dB or greater difference in hearing thresholds between the two ears at some audiometric frequencies or SRT). Clinical indicators of possible malingering may include lack of agreement between the PTA and SRT (±10 dB where the SRT is better than the PTA), inconsistent or exaggerated responses; SRT does not agree with the patient's prior ability to easily answer questions on the case history or instructions, or when the patient responds positively on virtually every question in the case history. Other "signs" that may warn the audiologist that the patient may exaggerate a hearing loss is if the reason for the visit is for the purpose of compensation or as part of a lawsuit.

The Stenger test involves the presentation of pure tone or speech stimuli (spondee words) to both ears simultaneously (dichotic or diotic listening). In theory, when tonal or speech stimuli are presented to the ears at the same time, with one stimulus louder in one ear, the ear where the SL is greatest will perceive the sound. For a pure tone Stenger test, a tone is introduced to the "better" ear at 10 dB above threshold and to the "poorer" ear at 10 dB below the admitted threshold. If the patient responds to the tones, the audiologist would know that he or she did indeed hear the sound in the better ear; however, if the patient fails to respond, this may indicate that the person is malingering. For example, at 1,000 Hz a patient has an admitted threshold of 20 dB HL in the right ear and 60 dB HL in the left ear. The audiologist elects to use the pure tone Stenger test to rule out malingering, and therefore, simultaneously introduces a 1,000 Hz tone to the right ear at 30 dB HL (10 dB above threshold) and to the left ear at 50 dB HL (10 dB below threshold). If the patient responds to the presentation of the tones, then the Stenger test is negative and suggests that the patient indeed has poorer hearing in the ear in question. If the patient fails to respond, then the Stenger test is positive and suggests a functional hearing loss in the poorer ear.

• How Are Tuning Fork Tests Utilized Clinically?

Tuning fork tests are rarely used by audiologists, but are used by otologists and otolaryngologists with greater regularity. If an audiologist does perform such tests, he/she will typically use the BC vibrator rather than a tuning fork to present the stimuli. This is because the stimuli being sent by the bone vibrator is clear of any distortion, is of a known and calibrated intensity level, and does not decrease in intensity over time.

Tuning fork tests used in audiology consist of the Weber, Rinne, Bing, and Schwabach tests. All of these examinations serve to identify the type or location of hearing loss. The Weber test is used to identify a unilateral hearing loss as conductive or sensorineural. A tuning fork (usually 512 or 1,024 Hz) is placed at the midline of the skull on the forehead and the patient is asked to determine where he/she hears the sound. If the patient lateralizes the sound to the better ear, the test is suggestive of sensorineural loss in the poorer ear. If the patient lateralizes to the poorer ear, the test is suggestive of a conductive loss in the poorer ear. Individuals with normal hearing or with bilateral sensorineural hearing loss will lateralize to midline or will hear the tone in both ears equally. The Weber test may also be performed with the use of a BC oscillator as part of an audiometric evaluation. The Rinne test is also used to identify a hearing loss as sensorineural or conductive, and involves placing the tuning fork near the external auditory canal and on the mastoid process and asking the patient in which position the tone sounds loudest. If the patient reports that the tone is loudest when the tuning fork is placed on the mastoid process, then the test is suggestive of a CHL. If the patient reports that the tone is loudest when the tuning fork is held near the outer ear, then the test is suggestive of normal hearing or sensorineural hearing loss. The Bing test is used to determine if the occlusion effect exists when the patient's ear canal is closed off. The tuning fork is placed on the mastoid process while the patient's ear canal is alternately opened and closed by pressing on the tragus. If the tone is louder when the ear canal is closed, then the test is suggestive of normal hearing or sensorineural hearing loss. If the tone does not sound louder when the ear canal is closed, then the test is suggestive of CHL. The tuning fork test that is least commonly utilized is the Schwabach test, which is used to estimate AC thresholds of the patient by measuring the amount of time it takes for the patient to cease to hear a tone after the tuning fork has been struck.

Table 2.7 provides guidelines for interpretation of the most commonly used tuning fork tests: Weber, Rinne, and Bing.

Table 2.7 Interpretation of tuning fork tests

Tuning fork test	Outcome	Interpretation
Weber	Lateralize to better ear	Sensorineural loss in poorer ear
	Lateralize to poorer ear	Conductive loss in the poorer ear
Rinne	Tone loudest via bone conduction	Conductive loss
	Tone loudest via air conduction	Sensorineural loss or normal hearing
Bing	Tone louder with tragus closed versus tragus open	Sensorineural loss or normal hearing
	Tone same with tragus closed and tragus open	Conductive loss

● What Are Otoacoustic Emissions and How Are They Interpreted?

Otoacoustic emissions (OAE), commonly referred to as cochlear "echoes," reflect the active processes of the outer hair cells in the cochlea. Though some individuals have spontaneous OAE, most individuals do not. Evoked OAE, more specifically transient-evoked OAE (TEOAE) and distortion product OAE (DPOAE) are most commonly used in the clinical setting to objectively assess outer hair cell function. OAE provide direct information regarding inner ear status (absent in moderate to profound SNHL) and indirect information regarding middle ear status (absent in CHL), and are especially useful in newborn hearing screenings, determining sensory versus neural pathology, ototoxic monitoring, in cases of suspected malingering, and in patients who are difficult to test behaviorally. Present OAE do not mean that hearing is normal, as OAE only begin to decrease at hearing losses of ~30 to 40 dB HL[9]; therefore, OAE cannot be used to estimate audiometric thresholds. OAE are measured with a probe assembly placed in the ear canal consisting of two or three ports: one or two loudspeakers for introduction of the stimulus and a microphone to record the OAE in the ear canal. Measurement of OAE occurs through the use of time-locked signal averaging; therefore, a quiet test environment and quiet patient are important factors.

TEOAE are evoked using a click or toneburst stimulus, and the obtained response therefore represents outer hair cell motility in the frequency region surrounding 2,000 Hz for click stimuli and at the frequency of the toneburst for toneburst stimuli. TEOAE are typically analyzed based on amplitude, response reproducibility, and the signal-to-noise ratio (SNR), which are compared with normative data. Approximately 1,000 stimuli are presented at a level of 80 dB peak equivalent (pe) SPL, and the measured response amplitude is usually 60 to 70 dB below the presentation level 5. **Fig. 2.18** provides an example of a TEOAE (stimulus: 80 dB peSPL click) obtained from the left ear of a patient with normal hearing. This patient has present TEOAE as judged by the response amplitude of 18.9 dB; response reproducibility of 95, 97, 99, 99, and 96% at 1,000, 2,000, 3,000, 4,000, and 5,000 Hz, respectively; and, SNR of 13, 16, 22, 22, and 15 dB at 1,000, 2,000, 3,000, 4,000, and 5,000 Hz, respectively (as indicated in the box labeled response 18.9 dB in **Fig. 2.18**).

DPOAE are evoked by the simultaneous presentation of two pure tones (F1 and F2), which are separated in frequency by a ratio of ~1.2, and where F1 is presented at 65 dB SPL and F2 is presented at 55 dB SPL. The amplitude of the cubic distortion product (2F1-F2) is then measured in the ear canal and is considered to be the DPOAE. As a result, outer hair cell function at discrete frequency regions can be determined by varying the frequency of F1 and F2. The obtained DPOAE amplitudes are plotted similarly to an audiogram on a distortion-product (DP) gram, as can be seen in **Fig. 2.19**, where frequency is plotted on the x-axis and amplitude (in dB SPL) is plotted on the y-axis. The solid curve with the "x" symbols on the DP-gram corresponds to the amplitude (dB SPL) of the DPOAE plotted at each F2 frequency, and the lower curve with the triangle symbols are the levels of the measured noise floor (NF) in the ear canal. The two solid lines below

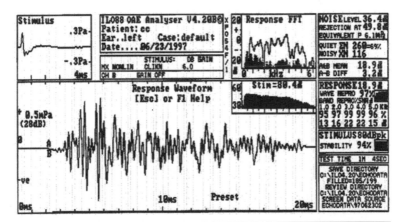

Fig. 2.18 Transient evoked otoacoustic emission (TEOAE) response from the left ear of a patient with normal audiometric thresholds.[8]

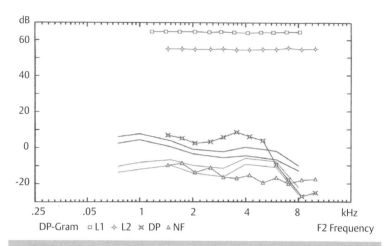

Fig. 2.19 DP-gram plotting the distortion product otoacoustic emissions from the left ear of a patient with normal audiometric thresholds. DPOAE were measured using an ototoxic monitoring protocol; therefore, emissions were measured from ~1,500 to 10,000 Hz.

the "x" symbol curve indicate normative values for the DP levels, and the two solid lines above the triangle curve represent the normative values for the NF levels. The curves for the squares and diamond symbols located at the top of the DP-gram are the measured stimulus level of F1 (65 dB SPL) and F2 (55 dB SPL) in the ear canal, respectively, and are used to monitor the probe fit throughout testing. Much like TEOAE, DPOAE are evaluated based on amplitude, reproducibility, and SNR, which are compared with normative data.

● What Is Electrocochleography?

Auditory evoked potential (AEP) testing measures the amount of electrical activity from the peripheral and central auditory nervous system in response to an acoustic stimulus. AEP measurement results in the generation of a waveform, with time (msec) plotted on the x-axis and amplitude (microvolts, μV) on the y-axis. Response parameters used in the interpretation of AEPs may include the latency of the response, waveform morphology, and amplitude, which are compared with normative data. AEP testing requires a relaxed patient state and uses time-locked signal averaging and filtering to improve the SNR and minimize test artifact from external (environment) and internal (patient) noise sources.

Electrocochleography (ECOG or ECochG) is one such AEP that measures the electrical activity generated in the cochlea and vestibulocochlear nerve (CN VIII). The components of this AEP are the cochlear microphonic (CM) potential, the summating potential (SP), and the compound action potential (AP) of the auditory nerve. Generator sites for ECOG components are as follows: CM—outer hair cells; SP—outer hair cells, inner hair cells, and organ of Corti; AP—afferent fibers of the distal eighth cranial nerve and spiral ganglion.[10] In ECOG testing, alternating polarity click stimuli at 85 dBnHL (dB normalized hearing level) are presented to the TE, and the response is recorded with the following electrode montage: an active electrode at the ipsilateral ear canal (or it may be placed on the tympanic membrane or promontory), a reference electrode at the vertex (or contralateral earlobe/mastoid), and a ground electrode on the forehead. This response occurs in the first 5 milliseconds following the onset of an acoustic stimulus, and the component parts are recorded on an electrocochleogram. ECOG test results are interpreted by calculating the summating potential:action potential (SP:AP) amplitude ratio, where a normal SP:AP ratio is considered to be less than 0.5 µV. **Fig. 2.20** illustrates a normal electrocochleogram.

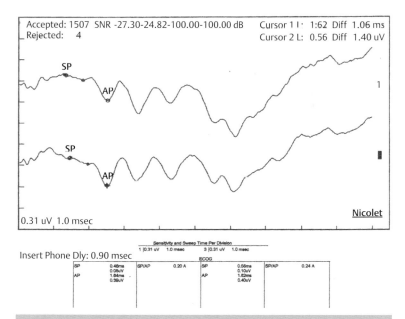

Fig. 2.20 Normal electrocochleography (ECOG) tracing: SP/AP = 0.08 µV/0.39 µV = 0.20.

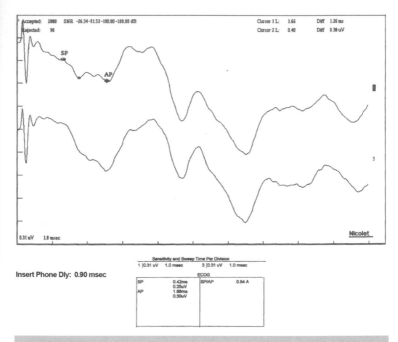

Fig. 2.21 Abnormal electrocochleography (ECOG) tracing: SP/AP = 0.25 µV/0.30 µV = 0.84.

ECOG is most commonly used in the differential diagnosis of Meniere's disease. In addition, ECOG may be used for enhancement of wave I of the ABR (AP of the electrocochleogram), intraoperative monitoring in an attempt to preserve hearing, and in the diagnosis of auditory neuropathy. In patients with Meniere's disease, the SP is enlarged and the SP:AP ratio is greater than or equal to 0.5 µV, as is illustrated in **Fig. 2.21**. It is important to keep in mind that other pathologies that may influence basilar membrane mechanics, such as perilymph fistula and superior semicircular canal dehiscence, will also result in an enlarged SP and, therefore, an abnormal SP:AP ratio.

What Is Auditory Brainstem Response Testing?

The ABR is a measurement of the synchronous neural activity of the auditory nerve and auditory brainstem in response to an acoustic stimulus. ABR testing utilizes click and/or toneburst stimuli that are introduced to the ear via an insert earphone, headphone, or BC oscillator. Electrodes placed at the vertex and on each earlobe (or mastoid) are used to record the ABR. The ABR waveform consists of five to seven vertex-positive peaks, which are generated in the first 10 milliseconds following stimulus onset and are labeled using Roman numerals. The ABR waveform involves multiple generator sites along the auditory nervous system: wave I—compound AP of distal portions of the auditory nerve, wave II—synchronous activity of the proximal auditory nerve, and waves III through V—multiple generator sites in the auditory brainstem.[11,12] Waves I, III, and V are the most prominent ABR components and the amplitude and latency of these waves are used in the interpretation of the ABR. The following ABR parameters are commonly used in interpretation: amplitude and amplitude ratio, absolute latencies of waves I, III, and V, interpeak latencies of waves I to III, III to V, and I to V, latency-intensity function, latency shift of wave V with stimulus rate increase, and the interaural latency difference of wave V. In addition, waveform morphology and replicability are important factors in ABR interpretation. **Table 2.8** provides normative information for a variety of ABR parameters used in interpretation, and **Fig. 2.22** illustrates both a normal and abnormal ABR tracing.

Table 2.8 Normative values for various parameters of auditory brainstem response interpretation

ABR parameter	Normal value
Amplitude	0.1–0.5 µV
Absolute latency at 75 dBnHL Wave I Wave III Wave V	1.6 millisecondsec ± 0.2 millisecondsec 3.7 millisecondsec ± 0.2 millisecondsec 5.6 millisecondsec ± 0.2 millisecondsec
Interpeak latencies Wave I–III Wave III–V Wave I–V	2.0 millisecondsec ± 0.4 millisecondsec 1.8 millisecondsec ± 0.4 millisecondsec 3.8 millisecondsec ± 0.4 millisecondsec
Latency-intensity function (50–70 dBnHL) Wave V	0.3 millisecondsec per 10 dB
Stimulus rate increase (21.1/s–67.1/s) Wave V latency shift	< 0.5 millisecondsec
Amplitude ratio Wave V/I	> 1.0 µV
Interaural latency difference Wave V	< 0.4 millisecondsec

Source: Data from Hood.[11]

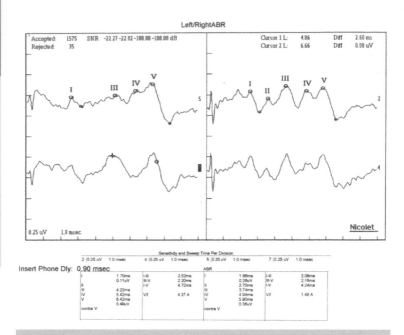

Fig. 2.22 ABR results from a patient with complaints of constant tinnitus in the left ear. ABR results were suggestive of retrocochlear dysfunction for the left ear and were normal for the right ear.

The ABR is clinically useful as a tool to estimate hearing sensitivity in patients who are difficult to test behaviorally, as a neurodiagnostic tool in an attempt to evaluate retrocochlear status (i.e., differential diagnosis of an acoustic neuroma), for intraoperative monitoring, and in newborn hearing screenings. When ABR testing is utilized for the purpose of estimating hearing sensitivity, the stimulus intensity is gradually decreased until the lowest level at which wave V is present can be determined. This level is defined as the ABR threshold and can predict hearing sensitivity within 5 to 20 dB.[11] Threshold ABR testing should use both click and toneburst stimuli to obtain as much diagnostic information as possible, because the click stimulus only estimates hearing sensitivity for a broad frequency range around 2,000 Hz.

When a neurodiagnostic ABR is performed, click stimuli at suprathreshold levels (≥ 75 dBnHL) are introduced to the TE and the interaural latency difference of wave V (often referred to as IT5) and the wave I to V interpeak latencies are analyzed and compared with normative data. In addition, stimuli may be presented at a slow (i.e., 21.1 stimuli per second) and fast (i.e., 67.1

stimuli per second) rate of presentation, and the amount by which wave V latency shifts is analyzed and compared with normative data. Criteria for referrals for otoneurologic ABR testing include unilateral and/or asymmetric sensorineural hearing loss, unilateral tinnitus, dizziness that is central in origin, poorer than expected WRSs, and significant acoustic reflex decay and/or elevated or absent ARTs. In making referrals for ABR testing, it is important to keep in mind that the degree and slope of hearing loss may affect the ability to obtain equivocal results. In general, ABR results in patients with PTAs greater than 80 dB HL at 2000 Hz and above may result in inconclusive results. Standard ABR testing is most sensitive at detecting medium and large tumors (> 1.5 cm). Another otoneurologic application of the ABR includes its use as a preoperative predictive indicator of hearing preservation following surgery for an acoustic neuroma. For example, the likelihood that hearing will be preserved in an acoustic neuroma patient with poor morphology and/or absent waveforms on an ABR preoperatively is small.

Common ABR patterns exist dependent upon pathology. Conductive hearing loss results in a prolongation of all waves, so absolute wave latencies are delayed, whereas interpeak latencies are within normal limits. Cochlear hearing losses may result in the absence or delay of wave I; therefore, the I to V interpeak latency may be reduced, and a steepened latency-intensity function may exist. Retrocochlear pathology may result in prolonged absolute latencies, prolonged interpeak latencies, interaural difference in the absolute latency of wave V, and poor morphology.

● When Is Ototoxic Monitoring Indicated and What Tests Are Involved?

It is well known that aminoglycoside antibiotics (i.e., streptomycin, gentamicin, neomycin) and platinum-based chemotherapeutics (i.e., cisplatin, carboplatin) have potentially ototoxic side effects, as does radiation therapy of the head and neck. Ototoxic monitoring is vital for patients who are taking such agents or undergoing cranial radiation therapy and typically involves both subjective and objective testing. Subjective measures include serial audiometry, with special attention to pure tone thresholds beyond 8,000 Hz (9, 10, 11.2, 12.5, 14, 16, 18, and 20 kHz), as well as tinnitus and noise surveys. Objective measures include tympanometry, acoustic reflexes, and DPOAEs. In addition, ABR testing may be performed in patients who are unable to provide accurate subjective responses due to a fragile health state.[13]

Ideally, baseline measurements should occur prior to the initiation of treatment or as soon as possible after treatment onset. The frequency of monitoring will be dependent upon the patient's drug regimen and is typically ordered by the referring physician. In addition, the patient should be advised to immediately report an onset of or significant change in hearing loss, tinnitus, or dizziness so that monitoring audiometry may be performed to confirm any ototoxic effects. Reporting of each serial audiogram is immediately communicated to the referring physician, with special note of significant threshold shifts when compared with the baseline. According to American Speech-Language-Hearing Association guidelines,[14] a significant threshold shift is defined as one of the following: a ≥ 20 dB decrease at one frequency, a ≥ 10 dB decrease at two adjacent frequencies, or loss of response at three consecutive frequencies. It is imperative that patients in an ototoxic monitoring program be properly counseled regarding the importance of hearing protection when exposed to loud noise and/ or the avoidance of loud noise, as noise can have a synergistic effect on hearing loss in patients taking ototoxic agents.

● What Is Cochlear Hydrops Analysis Masking Procedure?

CHAMP testing, which stands for cochlear hydrops analysis masking procedure, is utilized for differential diagnosis of Meniere's disease. Because Meniere's disease alters the mechanics of the basilar membrane and the way in which the cochlea processes auditory information, it is believed that low-frequency masking noise is less effective at masking higher frequency regions of the cochlea.[15] CHAMP testing uses the same electrode montage of standard ABR testing while click stimuli are delivered to the ear in the presence of high-pass pink noise with varying cutoff frequencies, identically to the stacked ABR protocol. In patients with Meniere's disease, wave V fails to increase in latency with the continual introduction of greater amounts of low-frequency energy in the masking noise, whereas in non-Meniere's patients, wave V increases in latency as greater low-frequency content is included in the masking noise. **Fig. 2.23** illustrates a CHAMP response in a patient with right Meniere's disease. The left ear response was within normal limits, as wave V latency increased significantly as the spectrum of the masking noise was broadened; however, the right ear response was abnormal, as wave V latency failed to shift significantly.

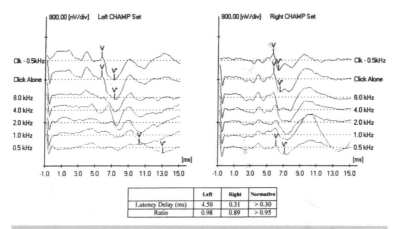

	Left	Right	Normative
Latency Delay (ms)	4.50	0.31	> 0.30
Ratio	0.98	0.89	> 0.95

Fig. 2.23 CHAMP tracing. A normal result was found for the left ear, as is noted by the shift in wave V latency; however, right ear results were abnormal, as wave V latency shift was not significant.

References

1. American National Standards Institute. Specification for Audiometers (S3.6–2010). New York, NY: Acoustical Society of America; 2010
2. American National Standards Institute. Specifications for Instruments to Measure Aural Acoustic Impedance and Admittance (S3.39–1987). New York, NY: Acoustical Society of America; 2012
3. American National Standards Institute. Maximum Permissible Ambient Noise Levels for Audiometric Test Rooms (S3.1–1999). New York, NY: Acoustical Society of America; 2013
4. Roeser RJ, Clark JL. Clinical masking. In: Roeser RJ, Valente M, Hosford-Dunn H, eds. Audiology: Diagnosis. 2nd ed. New York, NY: Thieme Medical Publishers, Inc; 2007:261–287
5. Hunter LH, Sanford CA. Tympanometry and wideband acoustic immittance. In: Katz, J, ed. Handbook of Clinical Audiology. 7th ed. Philadelphia, PA: Wolters Kluwer Health; 2015:137–163
6. Hunter L. 20Q: Acoustic immittance-what still works & what's new. AudiologyOnline Web site. http://www.audiologyonline.com/E/23143/ 94573/4c60ba5c54bca8e9d5. Published September 2013. Accessed July 20, 2016
7. Prieve BA, Feeney MP, Stenfelt S, Shahnaz N. Prediction of conductive hearing loss using wideband acoustic immittance. Ear Hear 2013;34(Suppl 1):54S–59S

8. Shahnaz N, Feeney MP, Schairer KS. Wideband acoustic immittance normative data: ethnicity, gender, aging, and instrumentation. Ear Hear 2013;34(Suppl 1):27S–35S

9. Glattke TJ, Robinette MS. Otoacoustic emissions. In: Roeser RJ, Valente M, Hosford-Dunn H, eds. Audiology: Diagnosis. 2nd ed. New York, NY: Thieme Medical Publishers, Inc; 2007:478–496

10. Ferraro JA. Electrocochleography. In: Roeser RJ, Valente M, Hosford-Dunn H, eds. Audiology: Diagnosis. 2nd ed. New York, NY: Thieme Medical Publishers, Inc; 2007:400–425

11. Hood LJ. Clinical Applications of the Auditory Brainstem Response. San Diego, CA: Singular Publishing Group, Inc; 1998

12. Arnold SA. The auditory brainstem response. In: Roeser RJ, Valente M, Hosford-Dunn H, eds. Audiology: Diagnosis. 2nd ed. New York, NY: Thieme Medical Publishers, Inc; 2007:426–442

13. Fausti SA, Helt WJ, Gordon JS, et al. Audiologic monitoring for ototoxicity and patient management. In: Campbell KCM, ed. Pharmacology and Ototoxicity for Audiologists. Clifton Park, NY: Delmar; 2007:230–251

14. American Speech-Language-Hearing Association. Guidelines for the audiologic management of individuals receiving cochleotoxic drug therapy. ASHA 1994;36(3):11–19

15. Don M, Kwong B, Tanaka C. A diagnostic test for Ménière's disease and cochlear hydrops: impaired high-pass noise masking of auditory brainstem responses. Otol Neurotol 2005;26(4):711–722

3 Vestibular Evaluation

● Who Should Be Sent for Vestibular Evaluation?

Vestibular evaluation provides the physician with objective and quantitative information regarding the function of the organs of balance. In patients with symptoms of dizziness, imbalance, and/or gait abnormalities of unclear etiology, vestibular evaluation can be used to rule out or confirm inner ear dysfunction. When an inner ear disorder has already been identified, vestibular evaluation can help to determine the extent of damage to inner ear structures, provide important lateralizing information, and help determine site of lesion. Results of vestibular tests can also be used to customize physical therapy exercises, determine risk of permanent balance dysfunction following cochlear implant surgery, or monitor the effects of vestibulotoxic drugs.

● What Is the Computerized Dynamic Posturography Test?

Balance and mobility are complex tasks that involve the coordination of numerous systems working together in harmony. **Computerized dynamic posturography** (**CDP**) evaluates the patient's ability to use these systems both together and independently. During the test, upright balance function is assessed and the patient's functional limitations are determined. This is accomplished through a variety of tasks that attempt to simulate conditions encountered in daily life. Unlike video-oculography (VOG) and rotational chair tests, which look primarily at the horizontal vestibulo-ocular reflex (VOR), CDP is unique in that it attempts to evaluate the function of the vestibulospinal reflex in addition to visual and somatosensory cues. Furthermore, performance on CDP is influenced by input from the vertical semicircular canals and otolith organs.[1]

To perform the test, the patient stands on a force platform that is surrounded on three sides by an enclosure that blocks the patient's field of view. The force platform consists of two footplates supported by five force sensors that detect exertion from the patient's feet along the horizontal and vertical axes.[2] Results of the test can be used to quantify and differentiate impairment in the sensory, motor, and central systems, as well as aid in the rehabilitation of the patient.[3] It can provide insight regarding the current state of central compensation in patients with a unilateral peripheral vestibular injury or bilateral loss. Furthermore, the test can help identify patients suspected to have exaggerated symptoms.

● What Is the Sensory Organization Test?

During the **Sensory Organization Test** (**SOT**), the patient attempts to maintain balance under six different conditions that incorporate various combinations of support surface and visual surround motion. Effective use of visual, vestibular, and somatosensory inputs as well as appropriate sensory integration and an intact musculoskeletal system are required to perform optimally on the test.[3]

There are six SOT conditions with a maximum of three trials each (**Fig. 3.1**): **Condition 1**—the platform and visual environment are stable. The patient has access to all three inputs to maintain balance. **Condition 2**—the platform is stable and the patient's eyes are closed. The patient must rely on vestibular and somatosensory inputs. **Condition 3**—the platform is stable, but the visual surround moves in concert with the patient (sway referenced) providing a distorted visual input. This assesses how well the patient can disregard the false input from the visual system and utilize the two other systems. **Condition 4**—the surround is now stable but the platform is sway referenced. Under this condition, the patient relies primarily on visual and vestibular inputs. **Condition 5**—the platform is sway referenced and the patient's eyes are closed. The patient must rely primarily on vestibular input because somatosensory and visual inputs have been distorted. **Condition 6**—the platform and surround are both sway referenced. The patient must rely on vestibular input and ignore false visual and somatosensory inputs.

Following each SOT trial, an equilibrium score is calculated (**Fig. 3.2**). The equilibrium score represents the maximum amount of anteroposterior (AP) sway that occurred during each trial.[2] The highest possible score is 100 (which would be indicative of no sway) and the lowest possible score is a 0 (fall or step). The greater the amount of AP sway during the trial, the closer the score is to 0. If the operator marks the trial as a fall, the word FALL appears on the graph and that trial is scored as a 0.[2]

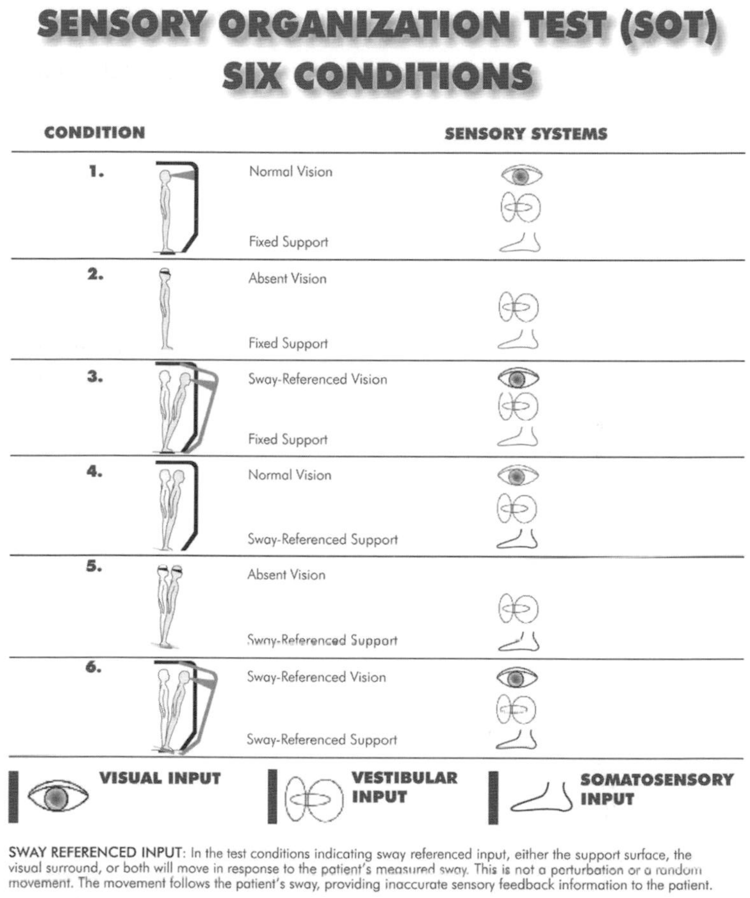

SENSORY ORGANIZATION TEST (SOT)
SIX CONDITIONS

CONDITION			SENSORY SYSTEMS
1.		Normal Vision	👁 👓
		Fixed Support	
2.		Absent Vision	👓
		Fixed Support	
3.		Sway-Referenced Vision	👁 👓
		Fixed Support	
4.		Normal Vision	👁 👓
		Sway-Referenced Support	
5.		Absent Vision	👓
		Swny-Referenced Support	
6.		Sway-Referenced Vision	👁 👓
		Sway-Referenced Support	

VISUAL INPUT   **VESTIBULAR INPUT**   **SOMATOSENSORY INPUT**

SWAY REFERENCED INPUT: In the test conditions indicating sway referenced input, either the support surface, the visual surround, or both will move in response to the patient's measured sway. This is not a perturbation or a random movement. The movement follows the patient's sway, providing inaccurate sensory feedback information to the patient.

Fig. 3.1 Sensory organization test—six conditions. The patient stands on a force platform with a visual surround on three sides to block the field of view. Each trial becomes progressively more difficult. The platform is fixed in the first three trials and sway referenced in the last three. The surround is sway referenced in trials 3 and 6. In trials 2 and 5, vision is denied. (This image is provided courtesy of Natus Medical Incorporated.)

The formula used to calculate the equilibrium score is as follows:

$$\text{Equilibrium} = \frac{12.5° - (\theta\,\text{max} - \theta\,\text{min})}{12.5°} \times 100$$

where 12.5 degrees is the normal limit of sway stability and θ represents the AP Center of gravity (COG) sway angle.[2]

Sensory Organization Test
(Sway Referenced Gain: 1.0)

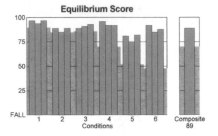

Equilibrium Score

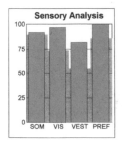

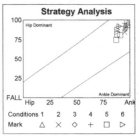

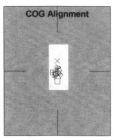

Data Range Note: NeuroCom Data Range: 20–59

Post Test Comment:

Fig. 3.2 Sensory organization test (SOT) comprehensive report in a normal subject. The equilibrium score illustrated by the top graph depicts the patient's performance on each trial of the SOT and is divided into the six SOT conditions. The composite score reflects the stability of the patient during the SOT test as a whole. The sensory analysis graph reflects patient performance when utilizing the different inputs to balance: somatosensory (SOM), visual (VIS), and vestibular (VEST), as well as the patient's ability to ignore conflicting visual input (PREF). Strategy analysis indicates the use of hip and ankle strategies to maintain balance. Scores approaching 100 indicate primary use of ankle strategy, whereas scores approaching 0 indicate primary use of hip strategy. COG alignment reflects the patient's center of gravity at the start of each SOT trial.

The score for each trial is displayed on a graph and compared with age-matched normative data within the system. Scores that exceed the shaded area on the graph are considered to be within normal limits and appear as a green bar on the graph. Those scores falling within the shaded area are considered outside normal limits and appear as a red bar. A composite equilibrium score is also calculated. "The composite equilibrium score is calculated by (a) independently averaging the scores for conditions 1 and 2; (b) adding these two scores to the equilibrium scores from each trial of sensory conditions 3, 4, 5, and 6; and (c) dividing that sum by the total number of trials."[2]

Specific sensory impairments to balance have been associated with various patterns of SOT performance (**Fig. 3.3**). Decreased SOT 5 and 6 is referred to as a **vestibular dysfunction** pattern.[3] These patients may have uncompensated unilateral or bilateral vestibular dysfunction. A look at the SOT raw data provides further insight regarding the extent of vestibular dysfunction. Patients with bilateral loss may demonstrate early falls on SOT 5 and 6,[4] which is indicative of a **vestibular loss** pattern while patients with unilateral vestibular function are more likely to exhibit late falls (**Fig. 3.4**). Decreased SOT 4, 5, and 6 is referred to as a **support surface dependence**

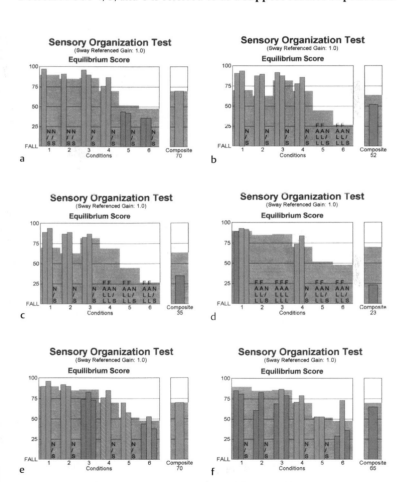

Fig. 3.3 Abnormal SOT patterns. (**a**) Vestibular dysfunction, (**b**) vestibular loss, (**c**) support surface dependence, (**d**) vision preference, (**e**) visual preference, (**f**) aphysiologic.

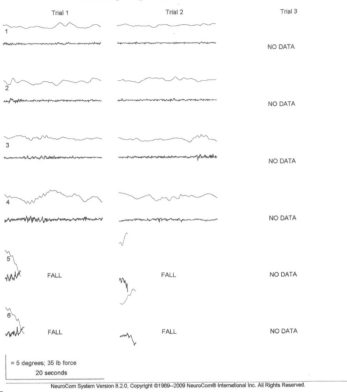

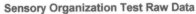

Fig. 3.4 The amount of time a patient is able to maintain balance before a fall differentiates vestibular loss from vestibular dysfunction. (**a**) Early falls during SOT trials 5 and 6 in a patient with bilateral vestibular loss and (**b**) Late falls during SOT trials 5 and 6 in a patient with unilateral vestibular dysfunction. (*continued*)

(somatosensory dependence) pattern and indicates impairment in the use of both vestibular and visual inputs to balance. Decreased SOT 2, 3, 5, and 6 is referred to as a **visual dependence** pattern. These patients may have impairment in the utilization of both somatosensory and vestibular inputs. Decreased SOT 3 and 6 is referred to as a **vision preference** pattern.[3] These patients may have impairment in the central adaptive mechanisms for suppression of conflicting visual input.[3] An **aphysiologic** pattern is characterized as one in which the patient performs better on the more difficult conditions or has great inter-test variability.[3] This may also present as a

Sensory Organization Test Raw Data

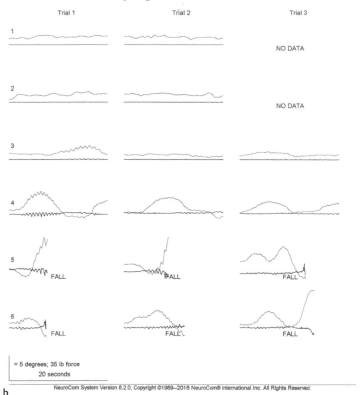

Fig. 3.4 (b) Late falls during SOT trials 5 and 6 in a patient with unilateral vestibular dysfunction.

global dysfunction in a patient in which observation prior to the test suggests a higher level of functional ability.

Results of the SOT may provide indications of aphysiologic performance. This may occur in several ways: (1) an improvement in postural ability on the more difficult conditions, (2) considerable inter-trial variability as seen in **Fig. 3.5**, (3) reduced scores on condition 1 when the patient did not appear to have postural or gait instability immediately prior to the examination, and/or (4) excessive lateral and/or circular sway patterns as seen in **Fig. 3.6**.[3]

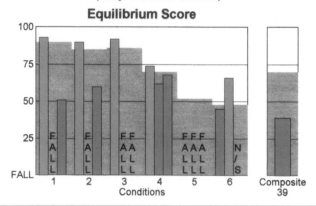

Fig. 3.5 Inter-trial variability on the sensory organization test.

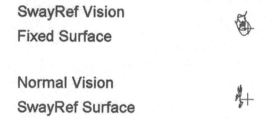

Fig. 3.6 Circular sway as seen on the raw data tracing of the sensory organization test in a patient with aphysiologic balance dysfunction.

● What Can Be Gained from Center of Gravity Scores and Strategy Analysis?

COG alignment appears as a scatter plot on the comprehensive report for the SOT and reflects the patient's COG at the start of each SOT trial[2] (**Fig. 3.2**). COG scores are useful in determining the patient's risk of falls. To remain upright, the body must be able to maintain its COG on a relatively small base of support. A person's limits of stability is defined as the maximum distance the body can lean in any given direction without losing balance. When the body is placed beyond its limits of stability, one must take a step or stumble to recover balance and avoid falling.[3] Therefore, a COG that is significantly eccentric reduces the distance the body can lean in that direction before exceeding the limits of stability, thus placing the patient at a higher risk for falls.

Strategy analysis helps to determine if the patient uses ankle and hip strategies appropriately when performing balance tasks (**Fig. 3.2**). Strategy analysis scores range from 100 to 0. A score of 100 indicates exclusive use of ankle strategy, and a score of 0 indicates exclusive use of hip strategy.[2] Strategy analysis scores that lie between the two extremes indicate a combination of the two strategies was used.[2] The strategy analysis is calculated by the following formula:

$$\text{Movement strategy} = \frac{1 - (Sh_{MAX} - Sh_{MIN})}{25} \times 100^{2}$$

In this formula, 25 lb is the "difference measured between the greatest shear force (Sh_{MAX}) and the lowest shear force (Sh_{MIN}) generated by a test group of normal subjects who used only hip sway to balance on a narrow beam (Nashner, unpublished data)."[2] Ankle strategy is most appropriate for small adjustments to the center of gravity such as those that occur when the support surface is firm and movement is slow. Hip strategies are more effective with rapid movements or when COG approaches the limits of stability.[3]

● What Is the Sensory Analysis Graph?

The sensory analysis graph is based on the average equilibrium scores of specific paired SOT conditions. It is designed to aid in the interpretation of how well the patient uses somatosensory, visual, and vestibular inputs as well as his or her ability to ignore conflicting visual input (**Fig. 3.2**).

● What Is the Motor Control Test?

The **motor control test** evaluates automatic motor reflex responses to sudden, unexpected forward and backward translations of the support surface.[2] The amplitude of the translations is determined by the individual patient's height. Three consecutive trials of small, medium, and large translations are recorded for both backward and forward perturbations. A score is determined for latency (msec), weight symmetry (%), and amplitude scaling (**Fig. 3.7**).

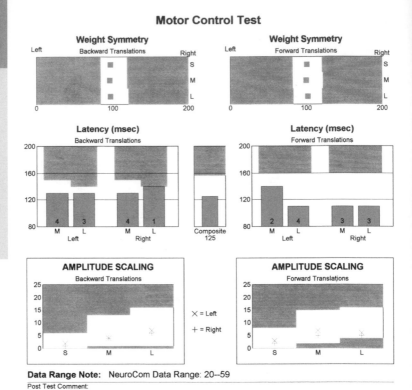

Fig. 3.7 Motor control test results in a normal subject. Weight symmetry indicates the percentage of body weight placed on each leg during small, medium, and large translations of the platform. Latency indicates the time lapse between onset of platform translation and the automatic postural response. Amplitude scaling indicates the strength of the response.

Latency refers to the time it takes for the automatic postural response to occur following the onset of platform translation. Latencies are calculated for each leg and each translation and are valuable for identifying motor system abnormalities.[5] Prolonged latencies imply dysfunction in any one or a combination of the components which comprise the long-loop automatic motor system and are most often associated with central and/or peripheral nervous system lesions[3,5] (e.g., multiple sclerosis/peripheral neuropathy).

Weight symmetry refers to the percentage of body weight that is placed on each individual leg during the motor control test.[3] Amplitude scaling provides indication of the strength of the postural response.[3]

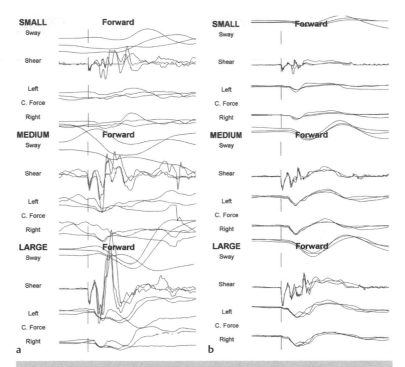

Fig. 3.8 Motor control test raw data. (**a**) Response tracings are inconsistent and reflect a voluntary component. (**b**) Response tracings obtained on a patient with normal function or true pathology.

Examination of motor control test raw data may provide further insight when an aphysiologic cause is suspected. A voluntary component is suspected when response tracings vary dramatically from one trial to the next, or when responses to small translations are large and highly variable[3] (**Fig. 3.8**). Aphysiologic patterns may occur in patients who are either highly anxious or deliberately exaggerating sway.[3]

● What Is the Adaptation Test?

As described by Nashner,[3] "The adaptation test assesses the ability to balance on irregular surfaces by suppressing automatic reactions to surface perturbations when they are disruptive to our stability." During the adaptation test, the patient attempts to maintain his or her balance during identical sequences of five toes-up and five toes-down rotations of the platform.[3] The amplitude of the patient's sway is measured immediately

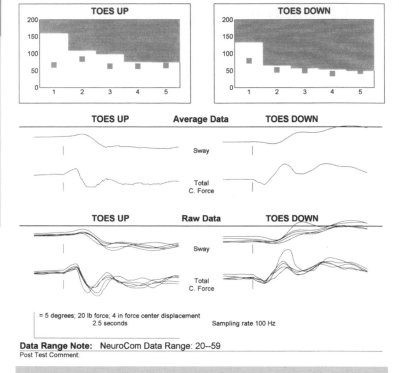

Fig. 3.9 Adaptation test results in a normal subject.

following each surface rotation (**Fig. 3.9**). Measurements indicate how well the patient is able to utilize adaptive mechanisms to enhance stability.[5]

● What Are the Clinical Applications of the Computerized Dynamic Posturography Test?

CDP may provide useful information in patients with case histories that indicate a history of falls, disequilibrium, postural instability, gait abnormalities, chronic symptoms indicating inadequate compensation, vertigo or dizziness of unknown etiology, or when a non-organic cause is suspected. Results from CDP may also be applied to the development and monitoring of vestibular rehabilitation.[2]

● What Are the Limitations of the Computerized Dynamic Posturography Test?

CDP does not indicate specific pathology but rather provides a quantitative assessment of the patient's functional limitations. CDP cannot be performed on every patient. Physical requirements for the test include a minimum weight of 40 lb, minimum height of 30", and the ability to stand unassisted for more than 2 to 3 minutes.[2] It should be noted that some of the SOT trials cannot be completed if the patient is blind.

● What Is Video-Oculography?

Video-oculography (**VOG**), also known as **videonystagmography (VNG)**, is the most frequently ordered test in the dizziness and balance laboratory. Sometimes still referred to as **electronystagmography** or **ENG**, VOG utilizes video rather than electrode recording (**Fig. 3.10**). VOG is a combination of

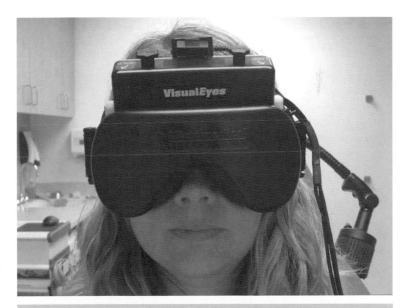

Fig. 3.10 Video-oculography goggles. Infrared cameras track the movement of the patient's eyes. A removable cover is used to allow testing with and without fixation.

tests that assess ocular motor function and the horizontal VOR. The test helps to differentiate between peripheral and central causes of dizziness and imbalance as well as provides important lateralization cues. The VOG test battery may include, but is not limited to, the following subtests: random saccades, horizontal and/or vertical smooth pursuit, spontaneous nystagmus with and without fixation, gaze nystagmus with and without fixation, post-headshake, positional/positioning tests, bithermal calorics, and fixation suppression.

● How Are Abnormalities on Saccades Interpreted?

The **random saccade test** assesses velocity (degrees/second), accuracy (%), and latency (msec) of the eyes as they fixate upon alternating targets. Abnormalities on saccades are a central finding but may also be caused by factors such as inattention, age, visual acuity, or medication effect[6] (**Fig. 3.11**).

● How Are Pursuit Abnormalities Significant?

For the **smooth pursuit test**, the patient is asked to follow a target with his or her eyes as it moves in the horizontal or vertical plane. Abnormal findings on pursuit include saccadic or absent smooth pursuit and are considered a central finding (**Fig. 3.12**). Other factors that may cause abnormal findings on pursuit include the patient's age, visual acuity, vigilance, and medication effect.[7]

● When Is Spontaneous Nystagmus Significant and What Does It Mean?

Spontaneous nystagmus is measured first with the patient staring at a target directly in front of him or her and then with fixation denied. Spontaneous nystagmus is considered abnormal when the slow component velocity exceeds 6 degrees/second.[8] Characteristics of the nystagmus can help determine its origin.

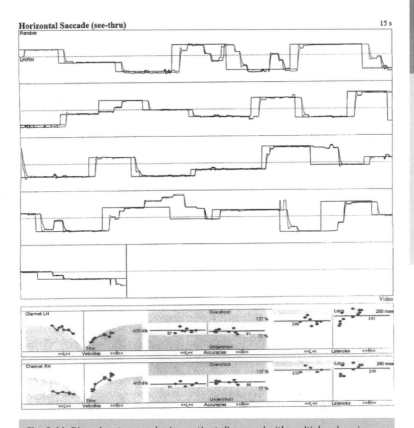

Fig. 3.11 Disconjugate saccades in a patient diagnosed with multiple sclerosis. Note the difference in left and right velocities.

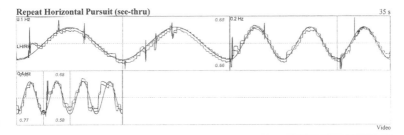

Fig. 3.12 Saccadic pursuit in a patient with central pathology.

Spontaneous nystagmus of **peripheral** origin is horizontal and becomes more pronounced when visual fixation is denied. The nystagmus is usually direction fixed. Alexander's law[9] states that spontaneous nystagmus due to a vestibular lesion will intensify with gaze in the direction of the fast phase and will diminish with gaze in the direction of the slow phase. Alexander classified the nystagmus by its intensity and direction. Nystagmus that is only visible when gazing in the direction of the fast phase is considered first-degree nystagmus.[9] The nystagmus is more intense with second-degree nystagmus and is visible when the eyes are in the neutral position as well as when gazing in the direction of the nystagmus.[9] The nystagmus is most intense in third-degree nystagmus and is present when gazing in all directions.[9] Patients with acute unilateral vestibular dysfunction may go through all three classifications as central compensation occurs.

Spontaneous nystagmus of central origin usually has a prominent vertical component, does not improve with fixation, and is accompanied with less vertigo than peripheral nystagmus.[10] Furthermore, central nystagmus often changes directions when gaze is directed away from the fast phase.[10]

● What Is the Significance of Gaze Nystagmus?

For the **gaze nystagmus test**, the patient is asked to hold the eyes in several eccentric positions first while staring at a target and then with fixation denied. Nystagmus that occurs only when the eyes are held in certain eccentric positions is referred to as gaze-evoked nystagmus. Gaze-evoked nystagmus is a central finding but may also be caused by alcohol or medication effect.[11,12]

● What Does Post-headshake Nystagmus Indicate?

The **post-headshake test** is useful for detecting asymmetry in vestibular tone and/or velocity storage.[6] For this test, the examiner rapidly shakes the patient's head in the plane of the horizontal canal for 10 to 20 seconds. Following headshake, the eyes are observed for any resultant nystagmus. Horizontal post-headshake nystagmus indicates a unilateral vestibular lesion and usually beats toward the stronger side.[13] In some instances, headshake nystagmus may beat toward the side of an irritative lesion as is sometimes seen in patients with Ménière's disease.[13] A vertical nystagmus that results from horizontal headshake is indicative of a central vestibular lesion.[6]

● What Do Positional/Positioning Tests Indicate?

Positional nystagmus is induced by holding the head in a specific position. To test for positional nystagmus, movement of the patient's eyes is observed while the patient holds the head and body in each position. Typical positions evaluated are the upright, supine, right ear-down, and left ear-down positions. Each position is maintained for a minimum of 30 seconds.[14] Positional nystagmus is considered abnormal if it exceeds 6 degrees/second in a single position and may be of peripheral or central origin.[10]

Positioning nystagmus is tested using the **Dix–Hallpike maneuver**.[15] The maneuver is performed by first turning the patient's head 45 degrees to the left or right while the patient is seated on the examining table. The examiner then assists the patient as he or she quickly moves into a reclined position with the head tilted back at a 30-degree angle while at the same time carefully supporting the patient's neck. The patient remains in this position for at least 60 seconds or until the response diminishes before rising back to the upright position. The maneuver is repeated with the head turned 45 degrees in the opposite direction.

The Dix–Hallpike maneuver is most sensitive when the patient is denied visual fixation although the torsional component is not suppressed by vision. The use of VOG or Frenzel lenses allows the examiner to directly observe the nystagmus elicited by the maneuver while fixation is denied. Diagnosis of **benign paroxysmal positional vertigo** (**BPPV**) can be made through the observation of the patient's nystagmus during the maneuver (**Fig. 3.13**). Diagnostic indicators include the latency (sec), duration (sec), and direction (rightward, leftward, upward, downward) of the nystagmus as well as fatigability with repeated provocation, the sensation of vertigo, and in some patients a reversal upon rising to a seated position.[14] It is characterized by its brief (2–15 sec) onset latency and subjective complaints of vertigo that typically last less than 30 seconds.[14]

BPPV is likely the most common cause of vertigo in the general population. In a study conducted in Germany, the 1-year incidence of BPPV was estimated to be as high as 0.6%.[16] Although it is confirmed by a positive finding on the

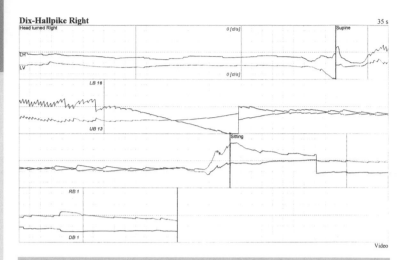

Dix-Hallpike Right   35 s

Fig. 3.13 The nystagmus response recorded during a right Dix-Hallpike maneuver in a patient with right posterior canal BPPV.

Dix–Hallpike maneuver, diagnosis is based primarily upon patient history. The patient will typically describe brief episodes of vertigo that occur with changes in head position such as rolling over in bed or looking up to a shelf.

There are multiple forms of BPPV. Observation of the nystagmus during the Dix–Hallpike maneuver provides insight regarding which semicircular canal is affected and whether it is due to **cupulolithiasis** or **canalithiasis**. Posterior canal canalithiasis is the most common form of BPPV, occurring in ~90% of cases.[14] It is characterized by an upbeating torsional geotropic nystagmus with the affected ear down.

BPPV in the horizontal canal is usually geotropic beating toward the under-most ear and is observed as a purely horizontal nystagmus. In this form, the debris is located in the affected ear down. At times, the nystagmus caused by lateral canal BPPV can be equivocal in both the right ear and left ear down positions making it difficult to determine where the debris is located. In these cases, the "**bow and lean test**" (**BLT**) can be a useful mea-sure.[17,18] Before performing the BLT, one must first identify if the nystagmus is geotropic (canalithiasis type) or ageotropic (cupulolithiasis type). While in the seated position, the patient is instructed to "bow" tilting their head downward over 90 degrees and then "lean" tilting their head upward over 45 degrees. The ear containing otolithic debris can then be identified as the same direction as "bowing" nystagmus in the canalithiasis type or in the same direction as "leaning" nystagmus in the cupulolithiasis type.[17]

Due to anatomical reasons, anterior canal BPPV is quite rare. It appears as an ageotropic downbeat nystagmus with the head hanging (affected ear up)[14] (**Table 3.1**). Recently, a variant of posterior canal BPPV has been identified with nystagmus similar to that expected from the anterior canal. In these cases, the debris is localized in the nonampullary arm of the posterior canal (affected ear down) and near the common crus.[19] This newly identified form of BPPV has been named "**apogeotropic posterior canal BPPV.**"[19,20]

There are two theories regarding the cause of BPPV. Cupulolithiasis was the first of the two theories to emerge. Described by Schucknecht in 1969, it is based upon his postmortem studies on patients diagnosed with BPPV. Schucknecht suggested that a deposit of dense particles (likely otoconia) lying on the cupula resulted in the structure becoming abnormally sensitive to gravitational force.[21] In cupulolithiasis, the otoconia remain attached to the cupula. The increased mass of the cupula results in vertigo and nystagmus, which occur immediately upon moving into the provoking position and persist until the patient changes position.[22]

The mechanics of cupulolithiasis do not agree with the latency and duration of symptoms seen in the majority of patients. It is for this reason that researchers were quick to question the theory. The theory of canalithiasis more readily explains the classic symptoms of BPPV. The theory of canalithiasis suggests that the otoconia/debris is free floating in the semicircular canal. As the head moves into the provoking position, the otoconia travels through the semicircular canal causing a hydrodynamic effect.[23] The movement of the endolymph stimulates the cupula causing symptoms of vertigo and nystagmus, which have a brief onset latency and usually diminish within 60 seconds. Furthermore, the response typically fatigues with repeated provocation.

Table 3.1 Distinguishing characteristics of benign paroxysmal positional vertigo (BPPV) by affected canal

	Posterior canal	**Horizontal canal**	**Anterior canal**
Incidence	Common, ~90% of cases (Gianoli and Smullen 2008)	Rare, ~6–8% of cases (Gianoli and Smullen 2008)	Rare, < 1% of cases (Gianoli and Smullen 2008)
Nystagmus	Geotropic rotary with a strong upward beating component	Horizontal geotropic in the majority of cases, ageotropic in ~10% of cases (Gianoli and Smullen 2008)	Ageotropic rotary with a strong downward beating component

● What Do Abnormal Caloric Test Results Indicate?

Caloric testing is often considered the most valued subtest of the VOG due to its ability to evaluate the responsiveness of the ears both individually and comparatively. The analysis of caloric symmetry is determined by each individual clinic's normative data and the mode of caloric irrigation. Options for caloric irrigation include open loop (water is irrigated directly into the ear canal), closed loop (water circulates within a balloon placed in the ear canal), and air (air flow is directed toward the tympanic membrane). Asymmetric caloric responses may denote a peripheral lesion. Absent responses may occur with bilateral vestibular loss, suppression, medication effect, or may also occur when there is a problem with temperature transfer.

Bithermal caloric irrigation is the most common method of testing. During caloric irrigation, the cupula of the horizontal canal should be oriented in a near vertical position to allow for optimal flow of the convection current created by the temperature change.[24] Typically, this is achieved by having the patient lie supine with the head elevated to a 30-degree angle. The ears are irrigated one at a time for ~45 seconds. The clinician may choose to irrigate with either the warm or the cool temperature first. Temperature settings should be verified at 44°C (warm) and 30°C (cool). During caloric irrigation, fixation is denied and nystagmus is recorded using infrared video cameras (VOG) or through electrodes (ENG). The examiner should explain the procedure prior to irrigation and make the patient aware that he or she may experience some dizziness. The examiner must also give the patient an alerting task as soon as irrigation begins to see the resultant nystagmus build. These tasks may be individualized for the best outcome. Tasking and recording of the nystagmus should begin at the start of irrigation and continue until the nystagmus begins to diminish. Once the nystagmus begins to diminish, the examiner instructs the patient to stare at a target to evaluate the patient's ability to fixate. Prior to irrigation, an otoscopic examination is necessary to ensure that there is nothing in the ear canal that may interfere with temperature transfer and to note any structural abnormalities. Open loop irrigation cannot be performed on patients with perforated eardrums.

The acronym **COWS** (**c**ool **o**pposite **w**arm **s**ame) can be used to remember the expected direction of the nystagmus following caloric stimulation. Responses to cool irrigation should elicit a nystagmus that beats in the opposite direction of the ear stimulated. Responses to warm irrigation should elicit nystagmus that beats in the same direction as the ear stimulated. In some instances, the patient may be tested in the prone position in which case the opposite will be true (cool same, warm opposite).

The use of two temperatures during caloric testing is important for accurate assessment. This is most obvious in cases where a spontaneous or positional nystagmus is present. In such a case, it is possible to have caloric responses that are deceptively symmetric or absent. It is also important to remember that the use of two temperatures allows us to measure two different types of responses. Warm temperatures result in an excitatory response, whereas cool temperatures are inhibitory.

Following the caloric test, calculations are made to determine the symmetry of the caloric response and directional preponderance. In most VOG software currently used, this calculation is based on a 10-second window determined by the examiner as the peak of the response for each caloric irrigation. Unilateral weakness is determined using Jongkee's formula:

$$\frac{(RW + RC) - (LC + LW)}{RW + RC + LC + LW} \times 100 = UW$$

where RW represents the peak response for right warm irrigation, RC represents the peak response for right cool irrigation, LC represents the peak response for left cool irrigation, LW represents the peak response for left warm irrigation, and UW stands for unilateral weakness.[25]

Caloric testing can provide important lateralizing clues; however, information gained from the caloric test is limited. It assesses only the horizontal canal at only one frequency (~0.003 Hz). Furthermore, the caloric test cannot differentiate between labyrinthine and retrolabyrinthine disease.

● What Does It Mean If the Patient Fails to Fixate Suppress?

Immediately following the caloric test, the patient is instructed to fixate upon a visual target. Estimation of the patient's ability to suppress the response is determined by comparing the velocity of the eye movement once the patient is allowed fixation with the velocity of the eye movement prior to fixation.[25] The nystagmus response from caloric irrigation should suppress markedly when the patient is given a visual target. In the case of good eyesight, failure to fixate suppress is indicative of cerebellar dysfunction.[8]

● What Is Directional Preponderance?

A directional preponderance exists when the nystagmus response from caloric stimulation is significantly greater in one direction versus the other. Directional preponderance is calculated using the values determined for the peak velocity of each irrigation of the caloric test in the following formula:[25]

$$\frac{(RW + LC) - (RC + LW)}{RW + LC + RC + LW} \times 100 = DP$$

A directional preponderance may occur with both peripheral and central vestibular lesions.[6] It is most often present in patients who have a strong spontaneous nystagmus.

● What Are the Clinical Applications of Video-Oculography?

VOG provides an objective recording of ocular motor function and quantitative assessment of nystagmus. Findings on the various subtests may indicate central pathology or peripheral vestibular pathology. Observation of nystagmus during the Dix–Hallpike maneuver can aid in the diagnosis of BPPV. Caloric testing may provide valuable lateralization information.

● What Are the Limitations of Video-Oculography?

Physical abilities need to be considered before sending a patient for VOG testing. VOG requires that at least one eye has a trackable pupil. Blindness may further limit the testing that can be performed. Positional/positioning tests require that the patient is able to move from a seated to a reclined position. Furthermore, the patient must be capable of following directions.

● What Is the Rotational Chair Test?

Motorized rotational chair testing is a valuable tool in the dizziness and balance laboratory. Often used in conjunction with VOG to confirm a diagnosis and increase accuracy, it allows assessment of multiple frequencies of the horizontal vestibular ocular reflex (0.01–1.0 Hz)[26] and provides information on the function of the velocity storage mechanism. When compared with the caloric test, the range of frequencies tested by rotational chair is closer to that found in natural head movement (up to 5 Hz).[27,28] Furthermore, rotational testing is not affected by the physical features of the ear[29] and is generally well tolerated by patients.

During the test, the patient is seated upright and secured to the chair with the head tilted downward 30 degrees to allow maximum stimulation of the horizontal semicircular canals. Eye movements are recorded using electrodes or infrared cameras. Use of restraints is necessary to prevent head slippage and avoid risk of injury. The chair is situated inside an enclosure to eliminate the influence of ambient light. Rotational chair testing can aid in differentiating between peripheral and central causes of dizziness and imbalance. In addition, it is a useful tool in determining the extent of peripheral lesions and provides information about the current state of compensation.

● What Is a Significant Finding on the Sinusoidal Harmonic Acceleration VOR Test?

Assessment of the VOR is performed using sinusoidal oscillation performed at multiple frequencies. The typical range of frequencies tested is between 0.01 and 1.0 Hz.[26] Ideally, the test is performed with the patient enclosed in a light-proof booth so that visual fixation is not possible. In addition, the patient is asked to perform mental tasking to avoid suppression of the response. Calculations are made for the gain, phase (degrees), and symmetry (%) of the nystagmus response (**Fig. 3.14**).

Gain measures indicate the strength of the response and are calculated by dividing the slow component velocity of the patient's eye movement by the slow component velocity of the stimulus.[26] A decrease in VOR gain occurs in both unilateral and bilateral vestibular loss (**Fig. 3.14**). Other causes of reduction in VOR gain include reduced alertness, suppression of the response, or conditions that restrict eye movement.[8] As central compensation occurs, gain values may begin to normalize.[30] VOR gain may be normal when the loss is restricted to the very low frequencies.

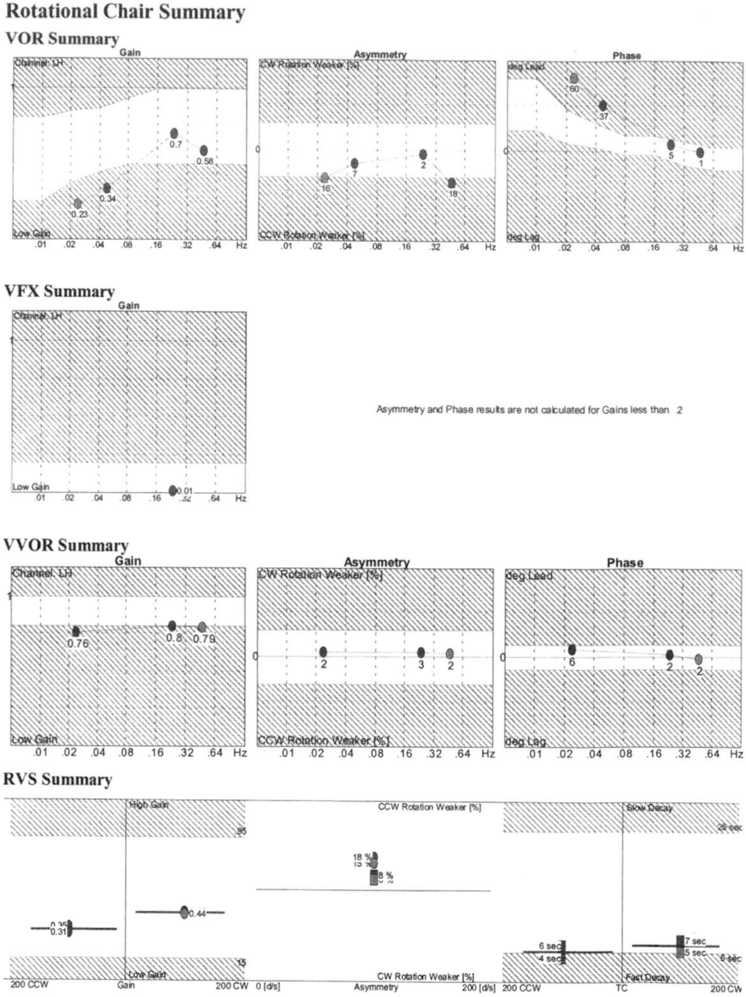

Rotational Chair Summary

VOR Summary

VFX Summary

Asymmetry and Phase results are not calculated for Gains less than 2

VVOR Summary

RVS Summary

Fig. 3.14 Rotational chair test summary in a patient with unilateral vestibular dysfunction. Note the reduced low-frequency VOR gain with accompanying phase lead and the reduced time constants (indicated by the rapid decay) on the rotational velocity-step (RVS) test summary. Abbreviations: VFX, visual fixation; CW, clockwise; CCW, counterclockwise.

Phase measures indicate the amount of time delay from the peak velocity of the stimulus to the peak velocity of the patient's eye movement.[31] Of the three calculations derived from VOR testing, phase is the most sensitive measure of peripheral vestibular function. An increase in phase lead is a strong indication of peripheral dysfunction (**Fig. 3.14**). Phase lag is considered a central finding.[8] Accurate measurement of phase requires a VOR gain which exceeds 0.2. Phase may remain abnormal as central compensation occurs.[30]

The symmetry of the response is the difference between responses during rightward versus leftward rotation.[31] Asymmetry in the VOR response implies imbalance within the system. This may occur with a static imbalance, as in acute lesions when a significant spontaneous nystagmus is present. Lesions that are dynamically uncompensated may also result in an asymmetric response.[8] Measures of symmetry have limited use in localizing site of lesion as abnormalities may be caused by either a unilateral weakness or an irritative lesion. Symmetry values normalize as central compensation occurs.[30]

● What Does It Mean If the Time Constant Is Decreased/Prolonged on the Step Velocity Test?

For the **step velocity test**, the chair is rapidly accelerated in a clockwise or counterclockwise direction until it reaches a predetermined velocity (between 60 and 180 degrees/seconds). Once the predetermined velocity is reached, the chair sustains that velocity for a period of 45 to 60 seconds.[8] Nystagmus is recorded while the chair rotates and is referred to as **per-rotary nystagmus**. Next, the chair is abruptly stopped and the **post-rotary nystagmus** is recorded for a period of ~30 seconds. The patient should be mentally tasked throughout the recording to avoid suppression of the response. The time constant is determined by calculating the amount of time it takes for the peak of per-rotary and post-rotary nystagmus responses to decay to 37% of peak value.[26] If the normal central velocity storage mechanism is intact, a time constant of greater than 6 seconds is expected. Reduced time constants are consistent with disabling of central velocity storage, which occurs with acute peripheral vestibular dysfunction (**Fig. 3.14**).

● What Is Velocity Storage?

Velocity storage is a central mechanism that allows for continuation of the raw vestibular response during sustained rotation. When the head is rotated, the cupula deflects in the opposite direction resulting in nystagmus. Due to the elastic properties of the cupula, it takes an estimated 6 seconds for the cupula to return to its resting position during sustained rotation.[6] The velocity storage mechanism is responsible for continuation of the nystagmus response for several additional seconds, which makes the VOR signal more useful during sustained rotation.

● What Does the Visual Vestibular Ocular Reflex Test Measure?

In this test of visual-vestibular interaction, the patient rotates in a clockwise or counterclockwise direction while viewing a stationary optokinetic stimulus.[8] Visual input contributes to the response most significantly in the lower frequencies and velocities.[27] For this reason, low-frequency visual vestibular ocular reflex (VVOR) gain may remain normal in cases of vestibular loss[27] providing further evidence that a poor VOR response is due to peripheral dysfunction and not a central ocular motor problem.

● What Does a Failure to Fixate Suppress Indicate?

This test evaluates the patient's ability to suppress the VOR when fixating upon a visual target. During this test, the patient stares at a laser light projected from the chair onto the wall in front of him or her. The chair and the light rotate together so that the light remains stationary in the patient's visual field. In the presence of good visual acuity, failure to fixate suppress the VOR suggests cerebellar or brain-stem abnormalities.[8]

● What Is the Optokinetic Nystagmus Test?

For optimal visual acuity, images must remain relatively stable on the retina. During head rotation, the VOR quickly reacts to stabilize the image. However, the VOR response is short lived, diminishing completely within 30 seconds. As the VOR response decays, the optokinetic and smooth pursuit systems supplement and eventually take over for the VOR to maintain the image on the retina.[6]

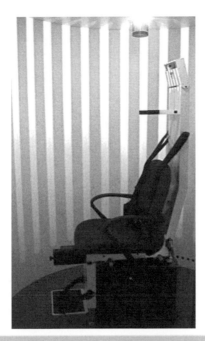

Fig. 3.15 Optokinetic stimulus as seen within the rotational chair enclosure.

Whereas the smooth pursuit system employs only the fovea, the optokinetic system utilizes the entire retina.[27] Therefore, to elicit a true optokinetic response, the stimulus must fill the entire visual field.[6] In the clinic, this is achieved by projecting stripes onto the wall of the rotational chair enclosure (**Fig. 3.15**). As the stripes rotate around patients, the eyes reflexively follow and patients begin to sense that they themselves are rotating. Abnormalities in optokinetic nystagmus (OPK/OKN) may indicate a central lesion.

● What Is the Dynamic Subjective Visual Vertical Test?

The otolith organs detect and respond to linear acceleration such as that caused by gravitational force. The response is an ocular counter-roll, with the eyes rotating in a compensatory direction.[32] An ocular counter-roll is also present following acute unilateral loss of otolith function. Static measurement of the **subjective visual vertical** (**SVV**) is obtained by instructing the patient to adjust an illuminated line or light bar to earth-vertical in an environment free of verticality cues such as while seated in a darkened enclosure or while looking into a hemispheric dome. During an acute loss, SVV measurements may illustrate a tilt of 10 to 20 degrees or more (patient's perception) toward the weaker ear.[33,34] In a period as short as a few weeks, central compensation occurs and the static SVV begins to normalize.[33,34] It is quite common for a patient's initial evaluation to take place after compensation has occurred when there may no longer be any outward visible signs of otolithic dysfunction.

Dynamic measurement of the SVV can reveal **utricular dysfunction** after compensation has occurred. There is some variability to how the test is performed. In our center, the patient sits upright in the rotational chair with his or her head and body secured in place (**Fig. 3.16**). The patient is instructed to manipulate a light bar to what appears to be earth-ver-

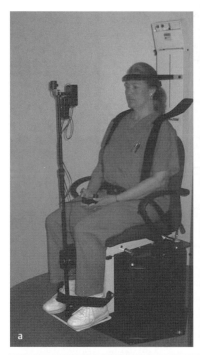
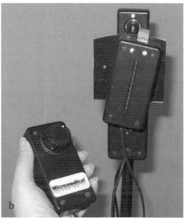
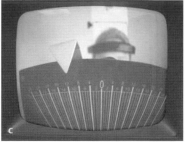

Fig. 3.16 The dynamic subjective visual vertical test. (**a**) Patient secured in the rotational chair with the light bar installed. (**b**) Patient's view of the light bar and the dial control used to adjust tilt. (**c**) Examiner's view of the light bar. Numbers indicate the degree of tilt.

tical under three conditions. Measurements are taken while the chair is static, during on-axis rotation, and during eccentric rotation. For dynamic measurements, the chair is accelerated to a constant angular velocity of 300 degrees/second. The utricles are stimulated by the resultant centripetal and tangential acceleration.[35] Measurements are taken after the chair has sustained this velocity for 1 minute to allow sufficient time for the response from the semicircular canals to extinguish. For each of the three conditions, the patient is asked to manipulate a light bar from both the right and left limits of the controller, to what appears to be earth-vertical (**Fig. 3.16**). This task is completed within a light-proof enclosure to ensure that the patient is not influenced by any outside reference. Degree of tilt is recorded by the examiner, and a comparison is made between static and dynamic measurements as well as the two eccentric conditions (left and right).

When rotated **on axis**, two normal functioning utricles will cancel each other out, resulting in minimal tilt. Minimal tilt may also occur in cases of bilateral dysfunction. A significant tilt following on-axis rotation may suggest unilateral dysfunction. Shifting the chair **off axis** allows stimulation of one utricle at a time. A study conducted by Nowé et al[36] investigating interutricular distance suggested that lateral displacement of 3.19 to 4.03 cm will align one labyrinth with the axis of rotation in the average Caucasian adult subject. The ear that is placed on axis receives minimal to no stimulation, whereas the eccentric ear is solely exposed to the acceleration of the chair.[37] If the eccentric ear is functioning properly, an ocular counter-roll should occur resulting in a tilt in the patient's perception of earth-vertical. Patients with impaired otolith function will demonstrate a reduction in tilt during rotation.

● What Are the Clinical Applications of the Rotational Chair?

Rotational chair testing provides dynamic assessment of the VOR and provides information regarding the patient's current state of compensation. Well tolerated by most and not requiring the patient to follow complicated instructions, rotational chair testing is often the test of choice in the pediatric population. In some cases, testing can even be completed while the patient is seated on a parent's lap. In patients whose caloric test results indicate a bilateral weakness, rotational chair testing can be used to verify caloric results and investigate the extent of dysfunction.

Rotational chair testing can detect peripheral lesions that are higher in frequency than those tested during the VOG. Standard caloric testing assesses the VOR at a frequency between 0.002 and 0.004 Hz,[26] whereas natural head movement occurs in a frequency range of ~0.1 to 5 Hz.[27,28] Typical rotational chair protocols test a portion of the frequencies occurring in natural head movement, specifically those between 0.01 and 1.00 Hz.[26] Due to the higher frequency range tested by rotational chair, it is sometimes used as a tool for monitoring ototoxicity.

● What Are the Limitations of the Rotational Chair?

With the exception of eccentric testing of utricular function during dynamic testing of the SVV, the rotational chair cannot test the ears separately and therefore is limited in its ability to provide important lateralizing information. In addition, claustrophobic patients may not be able to tolerate sitting within the enclosure and the test requires that at least one eye have a trackable pupil. DSVV may not be performed on persons who exceed the weight limitation of the rotational chair or those with medical contraindications (neck or back pain/injuries, history of stroke, etc.).

● What Is the Vestibular Evoked Myogenic Potential Test?

The **vestibular evoked myogenic potential** (**VEMP**) test is a valuable addition to the vestibular test battery providing information about the integrity of the otolith organs and the superior and inferior branches of the vestibular nerve. Development of the VEMP test was ignited in 1992 by Colebatch and Halmagyi[38] who described dependence of vestibular evoked potentials measured from the sternocleidomastoid (SCM) muscle on the integrity of the vestibular nerve and established a procedure to record them. The VEMP is a sonomotor response and can be elicited by several stimuli including air- and bone-conducted sound, head taps, vibration, and galvanic stimulation. Air-conducted 500 Hz tone burst sound is the most commonly used stimulus and is easily accessible through existing electrophysiological equipment. There are two types of VEMPs utilized clinically today; the **cervical VEMP** (**cVEMP**) response recorded from the ipsilateral SCM muscle and the **ocular VEMP** (**oVEMP**) recorded from the contralateral inferior oblique muscle.

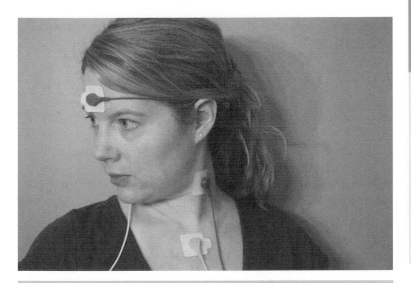

Fig. 3.17 Electrode array used to record cVEMP. The active electrode is placed on the belly of the ipsilateral sternocleidomastoid muscle, the reference electrode on the sternum, and the ground electrode on the forehead.

The cVEMP is a unilateral, inhibitory response arising from the saccule along the inferior vestibular nerve and recorded from the ipsilateral SCM muscle.[39,40,41,42,43,44,45,46,47] The air-conducted cVEMP response is obtained by presenting high-intensity clicks or tone bursts to the ear while the patient contracts the ipsilateral SCM. The response is measured via surface electrodes with the active electrode placed on the belly of the ipsilateral SCM. (**Fig. 3.17**)

The cVEMP response consists of two components, the first arising from vestibular afferents and the second arising from cochlear afferents.[39] The vestibular response is of primary interest and can be described as a short-latency alteration in electromyographic (EMG) activity appearing as a biphasic positive-negative wave (p13-n23)[39] (**Fig. 3.18**).

The oVEMP is a crossed, excitatory response primarily arising from the utricle along the superior vestibular nerve and recorded from the contralateral inferior oblique muscle.[47,49,50,51,52,53,54] The air-conducted oVEMP response is obtained by presenting high-intensity clicks or tone bursts to the ear while the patient fixates their gaze at a point 20 to 30 degrees upward and midline.[55,56,57] The response is measured via surface electrodes with the active electrode placed below the contralateral eye and midline or slightly off midline toward the lateral canthus to coincide with the belly of the inferior oblique muscle[58] (**Fig. 3.19**). The oVEMP response appears as a quadriphasic negative-positive (n1-p1 and n2-p2) complex (**Fig. 3.20**). The first negative

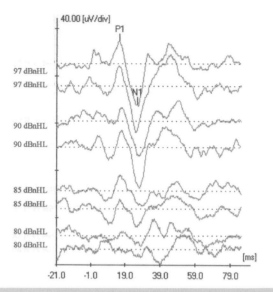

Fig. 3.18 cVEMP response in a normal subject. Responses were recorded down to a threshold of 85 dBnHL (decibels in normal hearing level). A behavioral reference, 0 dBnHL, is determined in the clinical facility by the average threshold response to the stimulus (click) in a small group of normal hearing young adults.[48]

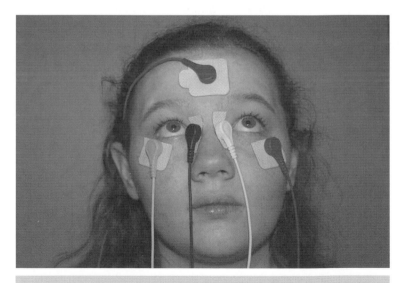

Fig. 3.19 Electrode array used to record oVEMP. The active electrode is placed beneath the contralateral eye near the belly of the inferior oblique muscle, the reference electrode on the contralateral side of the nasal bridge, and the ground electrode on the forehead.

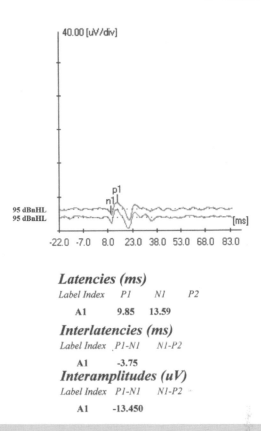

Fig. 3.20 oVEMP response in a normal subject. Only the first n1 and p1 of the quadriphasic complex are labeled here as they are of primary interest.

trough appears around 10 milliseconds representing excitation of the inferior oblique muscle and is thought to reflect activation of the utricle.[47,56]

● What Is a Significant Finding on the Vestibular Evoked Myogenic Potential Test?

Threshold (dBnHL), amplitude (μV), and latency (msec) measurements of the VEMP response have been studied for their clinical significance. Threshold measurements have proven useful in the detection of a third

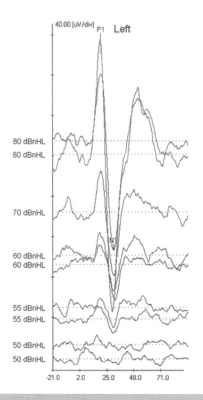

40.00 [uV/div] P1 Left

80 dBnHL
80 dBnHL

70 dBnHL

60 dBnHL
60 dBnHL

55 dBnHL
55 dBnHL

50 dBnHL
50 dBnHL

-21.0   2.0   25.0   48.0   71.0

Fig. 3.21 cVEMP response in a patient with superior semicircular canal dehiscence. Responses were recorded down to a threshold of 55 dBnHL.

window in the labyrinth, most often a **superior semicircular canal dehiscence** (**SSCD**). Due to increased compliance in the system, patients with SSCD may have abnormally reduced VEMP thresholds, 75 dBnHL or less[59,60,61] (**Fig. 3.21**). Reduced VEMP thresholds may also be seen in patients with other disorders including perilymph fistula and enlarged vestibular aqueduct.[59,62] The test's ability to detect SSCD is perhaps its clearest role.[63] It has been suggested that a combination of VEMP testing, computed tomography scan, and eye recordings may eliminate the need for surgical exploration to confirm the diagnosis of SSCD.[59]

The amplitude of the VEMP response has also been studied for clinical significance. Studies have shown abnormalities in amplitude can occur from several vestibular end-organ pathologies including Ménière's disease and vestibular neuritis, with amplitude asymmetry being the most common abnormality.[64,65] Amplitude measures, however, should be interpreted with caution. The amplitude of the cVEMP response has shown to be highly variable among normal subjects.[66] cVEMP amplitude is greatly influenced by the degree of muscle activation, stimulus intensity,[39,66] and has shown to decrease with age.[64] In the instance of SSCD, the amplitude of the cVEMP response is large but has limited diagnostic value due to the large amount of variance in normals.[59] Amplitude variability is not as great when recording oVEMP responses. Recent studies suggest that the air-conducted oVEMP provides the highest diagnostic yield in detecting SSCD due to significantly higher amplitudes when compared with normal subjects and requiring less time and effort than threshold measures.[67,68]

Due to high variability, the usefulness of absolute amplitude measures in cVEMPs is limited. Interaural amplitude asymmetry (IAA) is considered a more sensitive measure. Utilization of patient self-monitoring of EMG activity through biofeedback and the application of mathematical EMG amplitude normalization techniques appears to compensate for amplitude variability making IAA measures reliable.[69]

Latency of the VEMP response has also been studied and is considered a relatively stable aspect of the response.[70] Prolonged latencies have been reported in several central pathologies including multiple sclerosis.[71,72] Latency may also be prolonged with increased age.[64]

● What Effect Does Hearing Loss Have on the Vestibular Evoked Myogenic Potential Test?

The VEMP response is not impacted by sensorineural hearing loss.[39] This is in contrast to conductive hearing loss which can quickly abolish or attenuate the air-conducted VEMP response due to the decrease in stimulus intensity as it travels through the system. The presence of an air-conducted VEMP response in patients with conductive hearing loss is suggestive of SSCD.[60] Bone-conducted VEMPs are not affected by conductive hearing loss.[73]

● What Effect Does Age Have on the Vestibular Evoked Myogenic Potential Test?

VEMPs are well tolerated by children and can provide insight into the development of the sacculocollic reflex system as well as useful information about the maturation of the otolithic-ocular reflex, which is tied to the development of independent gait.[74] cVEMP responses can first be detected in newborns around day 2 to day 5, but maturity of the response does not occur until adolescence.[74] In particular, the latency of the p13 component differs significantly among children and adults and may be due to differences in the length of nerve fibers in the afferent/efferent pathways.[74] oVEMP responses are not identified in newborns; however, clear responses can be identified in children as young as 2 years and the response reaches adult levels around 3 years of age.[74]

Beginning in the sixth decade of life, the VEMP response in normals may be absent, amplitudes may be decreased, latencies may be prolonged, and asymmetry becomes more prevalent.[75] In the case of bilaterally absent VEMP responses in this age group, it can be difficult to determine if the absent response is due to impairment along the reflex pathway or is a result of aging.[76] A study by Piker et al[76] demonstrated changes in the frequency tuning of the VEMP response in older adults. This seems to be particularly true in the cVEMP response and is thought to be due to changes in the mass and stiffness of the end organs. In some older adults, the ideal frequency to elicit VEMPs appears to be 750 to 1,000 Hz.[76]

● What Are the Clinical Applications of the Vestibular Evoked Myogenic Potential Test?

Clinical applications of the VEMP test continue to be investigated. Currently, the VEMP has proven useful in the detection of SSCD. VEMPs can also provide lateralizing information and are useful in determining the integrity of the saccule, utricle, superior vestibular nerve, and inferior vestibular nerve.

What Are the Limitations of the Vestibular Evoked Myogenic Potential Test?

VEMPs are significantly impacted by age. As mentioned previously, VEMP responses are often absent or occur at alternate frequencies in adults 60 years of age or older. VEMPs require the cooperation of the patient and cannot be used with patients who are unconscious and are contraindicated in patients suffering from tinnitus due to the intensity of the stimulus.[45,73] VEMPs recorded from the SCM require that the patient be able to maintain adequate muscle contraction.[77] This may be particularly difficult for patients with weak neck muscles or muscle stiffness. oVEMPs require the patient to elevate his or her eyes, relax facial muscles, and refrain from blinking. Air-conducted VEMPs are abolished by external or middle ear disease.[77] Bone-conducted VEMPs can be used in patients with conductive hearing loss; however, current clinical equipment requires modification to provide the appropriate bone-conducted stimulus.[73]

What Is the Video Head Impulse Test?

The **video head impulse test** (**vHIT**) is an adaptation of the **bedside head impulse test** (**bHIT**) first introduced by Halmagyi and Curthoys in 1988 as a clinical sign of semicircular canal paresis.[78] The test is based on Ewald's second and third laws that describe the push–pull system of the paired semicircular canals and the relative inefficiency of the inhibitory response from the contralateral ear.[78] In the hands of the skilled examiner, the test has the ability to detect deficiencies of the VOR in all six semicircular canals.

How Is the vHIT Performed?

During the test, the patient wears a pair of lightweight goggles containing one or two high-speed video cameras that track the movement of the patient's pupil(s) and a gyroscope that detects the velocity, acceleration, and direction of head movement. To perform the test, the examiner administers unpredictable, high acceleration, low amplitude rotations of the patient's head in the plane of parallel semicircular canal pairs while the patient attempts to maintain visual fixation on a target placed 1 m in front of them. Head impulses in the horizontal plane assess the horizontal canals (**Fig. 3.22**) while diagonal impulses composed of equal components of pitch and roll, are the most effective way to evaluate the anterior and posterior canals[79] (**Fig. 3.23**). The impulses must be passive and their timing unpredictable. However, in the case of horizontal head impulses (and quite possibly vertical as well) predictability of the direction of head movement has little or no impact on test results.[80] For this reason, some examiners may choose to perform the impulses moving the patient's head from side to center as this technique is more easily tolerated by the patient and results in less neck strain.

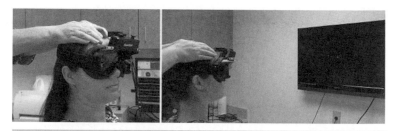

Fig. 3.22 Horizontal vHIT. The patient fixates on the target while the examiner quickly thrusts his or her head in the horizontal plane.

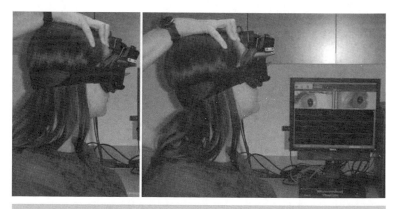

Fig. 3.23 Vertical vHIT. The patient fixates on the target while the examiner quickly thrusts his or her head in the plane of the anterior and posterior canals.

• What Is a Significant Finding on the vHIT?

During the head impulse, the examiner observes the patient's eyes to determine the presence of ipsilesional corrective saccades indicating that the patient was unable to maintain fixation on the target. The presence of covert and/or overt corrective saccades along with decreased gain values is indicative of a positive finding on the vHIT implying dysfunction in the ipsilateral canal (**Fig. 3.24**). Head and eye movements are recorded by the computer, analyzed, and displayed on a graph and gain values are calculated. Theoretically, a gain value of 1.0 is considered perfect and indicates that the eye movement is exactly equal and opposite head movement. Gain values below 0.7 are considered abnormal and are accompanied by covert and/or overt saccades displayed on the graph[81,82] (**Fig. 3.25**).

• What Are Overt and Covert Saccades?

Two types of catch-up saccades have been identified that occur as a result of VOR dysfunction during the head impulse test. Overt saccades occur

Lateral vHIT Video

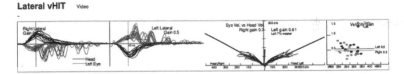

Fig. 3.24 vHIT responses in a patient with significant bilateral vestibular loss. Note the presence of both covert and overt saccades along with reduced gain values for both the right and left lateral semicircular canals.

Lateral vHIT Video

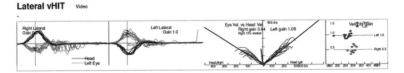

Fig. 3.25 vHIT responses 4 days post vestibular neuritis in the right ear. Note the presence of reduced gain and overt saccades for rightward head thrusts and the normal gain and absent saccades for leftward head thrusts.

after the head movement and are easily observed by the trained examiner. Covert saccades occur during the head movement with latencies as short as 70 milliseconds[83] and are almost impossible to observe by the naked eye. It is thought that covert saccades may be triggered, at least in part, by neck proprioceptors and are a sign of vestibular compensation.[84,85] In their observations of patients recovering from vestibular neuritis, Manzari et al[85] found that the temporal location of corrective saccades moved from overt to covert as patients began to compensate.

• What Are the Advantages of vHIT?

Prior to development of the vHIT, the bHIT was the only clinical means of assessing head impulses and relied on the examiner's ability to observe corrective saccades with the naked eye. While overt saccades that occur after the head movement are readily seen, covert saccades that occur during the head movement are hidden. Even in the hands of the most skilled examiner, the bHIT's inability to detect covert saccades makes the test's sensitivity moderate at best.[86] Covert saccades can be detected by scleral search coils, but they are not clinically feasible due to their high cost and patient discomfort. The ability of the vHIT to detect covert saccades is comparable to scleral search coils and can do so in a way that is both cost effective and comfortable for the patient.

• What Are the Clinical Applications of the vHIT?

The vHIT is well tolerated by most patients and is a quick, effective means of evaluating the function of all six semicircular canals individually. In acute cases of vertigo, the test can help the examiner to quickly distinguish vertigo caused by a cerebellar stroke from symptoms caused by a vestibular insult such as vestibular neuritis.[87] Once the acute insult has passed, the vHIT can be used to unmask central compensation which appears within the first few days.[88] The vHIT also provides insight into the state of compensation and thus may be used as a tool for therapists in their approach to rehabilitation.[89] When used in conjunction with caloric testing, it may be used to distinguish Ménière's disease from other etiologies. McCaslin et al[90] reported a pattern of ipsilesional abnormal caloric test results in the presence of normal video head impulse results in patients with "definite" Ménière's disease. In addition, the test is portable and can be used to test a wide range of ages including young children.[91]

• What Are the Limitations of the vHIT?

The vHIT requires high technical skill to perform. Assessment of the vertical canals is particularly difficult due to limitations in neck mobility and the high velocities necessary for evaluation.[91] The test requires patient cooperation. The patient must keep his or her eyes wide open and fixated on the target. Neck muscles must be relaxed to allow the examiner to turn the head passively and with an abrupt start and stop.[91] Adequate relaxation may be impossible in patients with unusually stiff necks. In addition, the patient must have at least one pupil that is trackable. Ocular abnormalities, such as scar tissue or permanent makeup, can cause confusion for the cameras and result in a recording that is too noisy to interpret.

To obtain accurate data, the goggles must fit tight and securely to the patient's head to reduce goggle slippage.[85] Even with the best fitting goggle some slippage may occur due to the flexibility of the skin.

It should be kept in mind that the vHIT provides different information than the caloric test and thus, serves more as a complementary tool than a replacement. The caloric test evaluates the system at a very low frequency of ~0.003 Hz. The vHIT is a test of high-frequency function, performed at frequencies up to 5 Hz,[92] and is within the range of natural head movement. Natural head movement occurs in the frequency range of 0.1 to 5 Hz.[27,28] The presence of normal vHITs in patients with caloric deficits is quite common. Studies have shown that a caloric deficit of close to more than 40% may be required before the deficit appears on the vHIT test.[88,89]

References

1. Furman JM. Role of posturography in the management of vestibular patients. Otolaryngol Head Neck Surg 1995;112(1):8–15
2. NeuroCom International. EquiTest system operators manual (version 7.04). Clackamas, OR: NeuroCom International, Inc; 2000
3. Nashner LM. Computerized dynamic posturography. In: Goebel JA, ed. Practical Management of the Dizzy Patient. 2nd ed. Philadelphia, PA: Lippincott Williams & Wilkins; 2008:153–182
4. Goebel JA, White JA, Heidenreich KD. Evaluation of the vestibular system. In: Snow JB, Wackym PA, Ballenger JJ, eds. Ballenger's Otorhinolaryngology Head and Neck Surgery. 17th ed. Shelton, CT: People's Medical Publishing House; 2009:131–144

5. Nashner LM. Computerized dynamic posturography. In: Jacobson GP, Newman CW, Kartush JM, eds. Handbook of Balance Function Testing. San Diego, CA: Delmar; 1997:280–307

6. Leigh RJ, Zee DS. The Neurology of Eye Movements. 2nd ed. Philadelphia, PA: F. A. Davis Company; 1991

7. Cass SP. Performing the physical examination: ocular motor examination. In: Goebel JA, ed. Practical Management of the Dizzy Patient. 2nd ed. Philadelphia, PA: Lippincott Williams & Wilkins; 2008:75–78

8. Shepard NT, Telian SA. Practical Management of the Balance Disorder Patient. San Diego, CA: Singular Publishing Group; 1996

9. Alexander G. Die Ohrenkrankheiten im Kindesalter. In: Pfaundler M, Schlossman A, eds. Handbuch der Kinderheilkunde. Leipzig, Germany: Vogel; 1912:84–96

10. Brandt T. Background, technique, interpretation, and usefulness of positional and positioning testing. In: Jacobson GP, Newman CW, Kartush JM, eds. Handbook of Balance Function Testing. San Diego, CA: Delmar; 1997:123–155

11. Hain TC. Interpretation and usefulness of ocular motility testing. In: Jacobson GP, Newman CW, Kartush JM, eds. Handbook of Balance Function Testing. San Diego, CA: Delmar; 1997:101–122

12. Bhansali SA. Medication side effects. In: Goebel JA, ed. Practical Management of the Dizzy Patient. 2nd ed. Philadelphia, PA: Lippincott Williams & Wilkins; 2008:43–60

13. Takahashi S, Fetter M, Koenig E, Dichgans J. The clinical significance of head-shaking nystagmus in the dizzy patient. Acta Otolaryngol 1990;109(1–2):8–14

14. Gianoli GJ, Smullen JL. Performing the physical examination: Positioning tests. In: Goebel, JA, ed. Practical Management of the Dizzy Patient. 2nd ed. Philadelphia, PA: Lippincott Williams & Wilkins; 2008:85–97

15. Dix MR, Hallpike CS. The pathology symptomatology and diagnosis of certain common disorders of the vestibular system. Proc R Soc Med 1952;45(6):341–354

16. von Brevern M, Radtke A, Lezius F, et al. Epidemiology of benign paroxysmal positional vertigo: a population based study. J Neurol Neurosurg Psychiatry 2007;78(7):710–715

17. Choung YH, Shin YR, Kahng H, Park K, Choi SJ. 'Bow and lean test' to determine the affected ear of horizontal canal benign paroxysmal positional vertigo. Laryngoscope 2006;116(10):1776–1781

18. Lee JB, Han DH, Choi SJ, et al. Efficacy of the "bow and lean test" for the management of horizontal canal benign paroxysmal positional vertigo. Laryngoscope 2010;120(11):2339–2346

19. Vannucchi P, Pecci R, Giannoni B. Posterior semicircular canal benign paroxysmal positional vertigo presenting with torsional downbeating nystagmus: an apogeotropic variant. Int J Otolaryngol 2012;2012: 413603

20. Califano L, Salafia F, Mazzone S, Melillo MG, Califano M. Anterior canal BPPV and apogeotropic posterior canal BPPV: two rare forms of vertical canalolithiasis. Acta Otorhinolaryngol Ital 2014;34(3):189–197

21. Schuknecht HF. Cupulolithiasis. Arch Otolaryngol 1969;90(6):765–778.

22. Herdman SJ, Tusa RJ. Assessment and treatment of patients with benign paroxysmal positional vertigo. In: Herdman SJ, ed. Vestibular Rehabilitation. 2nd ed. Philadelphia, PA: F. A. Davis Company; 2000:451–475

23. House MG, Honrubia V. Theoretical models for the mechanisms of benign paroxysmal positional vertigo. Audiol Neurootol 2003;8(2):91–99

24. Jacobson GP, Newman CW. Background and technique of caloric testing. In: Jacobson GP, Newman CW, Kartush M, eds. Handbook of Balance Function Testing. San Diego, CA: Delmar; 1997:156–192

25. Stockwell CW. ENG Workbook. Needham Heights, MA: Allyn and Bacon; 1983

26. Handelsman JA, Shepard NT. Rotational chair testing. In: Goebel JA, ed. Practical Management of the Dizzy Patient. 2nd ed. Philadelphia, PA: Lippincott Williams & Wilkins; 2008:137–152

27. Baloh RW, Honrubia V. Clinical Neurophysiology of the Vestibular System. 3rd ed. New York, NY: Oxford University Press, Inc.; 2001.

28. Jones GM, Milsum JH. Spatial and dynamic aspects of visual fixation. IEEE Trans Biomed Eng 1965;12(2):54–62

29. Honrubia V. Quantitative vestibular function tests and the clinical examination. In: Herdman SJ, ed. Vestibular Rehabilitation. 2nd ed. Philadelphia, PA: F. A. Davis Company; 2000:105–171

30. Desmond A. Vestibular Function: Evaluation and Treatment. New York, NY: Thieme Medical Publishers, Inc.; 2004

31. Micromedical Technologies. ENG, vorteq, and rotational chair user's manual. (version 4.5). Chatham, IL: Micromedical Technologies, Inc.; 1995

32. Halmagyi GM, Curthoys IS. Otolith function tests. In: Herdman SJ, ed. Vestibular Rehabilitation. 2nd ed. Philadelphia, PA: F. A. Davis Company; 2000:195–214

33. Böhmer A, Mast F. Chronic unilateral loss of otolith function revealed by the subjective visual vertical during off center yaw rotation. J Vestib Res 1999;9(6):413–422

34. Karlberg M, Aw ST, Halmagyi GM, Black RA. Vibration-induced shift of the subjective visual horizontal: a sign of unilateral vestibular deficit. Arch Otolaryngol Head Neck Surg 2002;128(1):21–27

35. Furman JMR, Baloh RW. Otolith-ocular testing in human subjects. Ann N Y Acad Sci 1992;656:431–451

36. Nowé V, Wuyts FL, Hoppenbrouwers M, Van de Heyning PH, De Schepper AM, Parizel PM. The interutricular distance determined from external landmarks. J Vestib Res 2003;13(1):17–23

37. Clarke AH, Engelhorn A. Unilateral testing of utricular function. Exp Brain Res 1998;121(4):457–464

38. Colebatch JG, Halmagyi GM. Vestibular evoked potentials in human neck muscles before and after unilateral vestibular deafferentation. Neurology 1992;42(8):1635–1636

39. Colebatch JG, Halmagyi GM, Skuse NF. Myogenic potentials generated by a click-evoked vestibulocollic reflex. J Neurol Neurosurg Psychiatry 1994;57(2):190–197

40. Halmagyi GM, Colebatch JG. Vestibular evoked myogenic potentials in the sternomastoid muscle are not of lateral canal origin. Acta Otolaryngol Suppl 1995;520(Pt 1):1–3

41. Uchino Y, Sato H, Sasaki M, et al. Sacculocollic reflex arcs in cats. J Neurophysiol 1997;77(6):3003–3012

42. Murofushi T, Matsuzaki M, Mizuno M. Vestibular evoked myogenic potentials in patients with acoustic neuromas. Arch Otolaryngol Head Neck Surg 1998;124(5):509–512

43. Li MW, Houlden D, Tomlinson RD. Click evoked EMG responses in sternocleidomastoid muscles: characteristics in normal subjects. J Vestib Res 1999;9(5):327–334

44. Todd NPM, Cody FWJ, Banks JR. A saccular origin of frequency tuning in myogenic vestibular evoked potentials?: implications for human responses to loud sounds. Hear Res 2000;141(1-2):180–188

45. Colebatch JG. Vestibular evoked potentials. Curr Opin Neurol 2001;14(1):21–26

46. Sheykholeslami K, Kaga K. The otolithic organ as a receptor of vestibular hearing revealed by vestibular-evoked myogenic potentials in patients with inner ear anomalies. Hear Res 2002;165(1–2):62–67

47. Iwasaki S, Chihara Y, Smulders YE, et al. The role of the superior vestibular nerve in generating ocular vestibular-evoked myogenic potentials to bone conducted vibration at Fz. Clin Neurophysiol 2009;120(3):588–593

48. Hall JW III. New Handbook of Auditory Evoked Responses. Boston: Pearson; 2007

49. Rosengren SM, McAngus Todd NP, Colebatch JG. Vestibular-evoked extraocular potentials produced by stimulation with bone-conducted sound. Clin Neurophysiol 2005;116(8):1938–1948

50. Chihara Y, Iwasaki S, Ushio M, Murofushi T. Vestibular-evoked extraocular potentials by air-conducted sound: another clinical test for vestibular function. Clin Neurophysiol 2007;118(12):2745–2751

51. Todd NPM, Rosengren SM, Colebatch JG. Ocular vestibular evoked myogenic potentials (OVEMPs) produced by impulsive transmastoid accelerations. Clin Neurophysiol 2008;119(7):1638–1651

52. Curthoys IS. A critical review of the neurophysiological evidence underlying clinical vestibular testing using sound, vibration and galvanic stimuli. Clin Neurophysiol 2010;121(2):132–144

53. Jacobson GP, McCaslin DL, Piker EG, Gruenwald J, Grantham SL, Tegel L. Patterns of abnormality in cVEMP, oVEMP, and caloric tests may provide topological information about vestibular impairment. J Am Acad Audiol 2011;22(9):601–611

54. Papathanasiou ES. The evidence is finally here: ocular vestibular evoked myogenic potentials are mainly dependent on utricular pathway function. Clin Neurophysiol 2015;126(10):1843–1844

55. Murnane OD, Akin FW, Kelly KJ, Byrd S. Effects of stimulus and recording parameters on the air conduction ocular vestibular evoked myogenic potential. J Am Acad Audiol 2011;22(7):469–480

56. Iwasaki S, Smulders YE, Burgess AM, et al. Ocular vestibular evoked myogenic potentials to bone conducted vibration of the midline forehead at Fz in healthy subjects. Clin Neurophysiol 2008;119(9):2135–2147

57. McCaslin DL, Jacobson GP. Vestibular-evoked myogenic potentials (VEMPS). In: Jacobson GP, Shepard NT, eds. Balance Function Assessment and Management. 2nd ed. San Diego, CA: Plural Publishing; 2016:533–579

58. Sandhu JS, George SR, Rea PA. The effect of electrode positioning on the ocular vestibular evoked myogenic potential to air-conducted sound. Clin Neurophysiol 2013;124(6):1232–1236

59. Watson SRD, Halmagyi GM, Colebatch JG. Vestibular hypersensitivity to sound (Tullio phenomenon): structural and functional assessment. Neurology 2000;54(3):722–728

60. Streubel SO, Cremer PD, Carey JP, Weg N, Minor LB. Vestibular-evoked myogenic potentials in the diagnosis of superior canal dehiscence syndrome. Acta Otolaryngol Suppl 2001;545:41–49

61. Brantberg K, Löfqvist L, Fransson PA. Large vestibular evoked myogenic potentials in response to bone-conducted sounds in patients with superior canal dehiscence syndrome. Audiol Neurootol 2004;9(3):173–182

62. Sheykholeslami K, Schmerber S, Habiby Kermany M, Kaga K. Vestibular-evoked myogenic potentials in three patients with large vestibular aqueduct. Hear Res 2004;190(1–2):161–168

63. Rosengren SM, Kingma H. New perspectives on vestibular evoked myogenic potentials. Curr Opin Neurol 2013;26(1):74–80

64. Zapala DA, Brey RH. Clinical experience with the vestibular evoked myogenic potential. J Am Acad Audiol 2004;15(3):198–215

65. Todd NPM. The origin of the ocular vestibular evoked myogenic potential (OVEMP). Clin Neurophysiol 2010;121(6):978–980

66. Lim CL, Clouston P, Sheean G, Yiannikas C. The influence of voluntary EMG activity and click intensity on the vestibular click evoked myogenic potential. Muscle Nerve 1995;18(10):1210–1213

67. Zuniga MG, Janky KL, Nguyen KD, Welgampola MS, Carey JP. Ocular versus cervical VEMPs in the diagnosis of superior semicircular canal dehiscence syndrome. Otol Neurotol 2013;34(1):121–126

68. Janky KL, Nguyen KD, Welgampola M, Zuniga MG, Carey JP. Air-conducted oVEMPs provide the best separation between intact and superior canal dehiscent labyrinths. Otol Neurotol 2013;34(1):127–134

69. McCaslin DL, Fowler A, Jacobson GP. Amplitude normalization reduces cervical vestibular evoked myogenic potential (cVEMP) amplitude asymmetries in normal subjects: proof of concept. J Am Acad Audiol 2014;25(3):268–277

70. Zhou G, Cox LC. Vestibular evoked myogenic potentials: history and overview. Am J Audiol 2004;13(2):135–143

71. Murofushi T, Shimizu K, Takegoshi H, Cheng PW. Diagnostic value of prolonged latencies in the vestibular evoked myogenic potential. Arch Otolaryngol Head Neck Surg 2001;127(9):1069–1072

72. Bandini F, Beronio A, Ghiglione E, Solaro C, Parodi RC, Mazzella L. The diagnostic value of vestibular evoked myogenic potentials in multiple sclerosis. J Neurol 2004;251(5):617–621

73. Welgampola MS, Colebatch JG. Characteristics and clinical applications of vestibular-evoked myogenic potentials. Neurology 2005;64(10):1682–1688

74. Young YH. Assessment of functional development of the otolithic system in growing children: a review. Int J Pediatr Otorhinolaryngol 2015;79(4):435–442

75. Welgampola MS, Colebatch JG. Vestibulocollic reflexes: normal values and the effect of age. Clin Neurophysiol 2001;112(11):1971–1979

76. Piker EG, Jacobson GP, Burkard RF, McCaslin DL, Hood LJ. Effects of age on the tuning of the cVEMP and oVEMP. Ear Hear 2013;34(6):e65–e73

77. Alpini D, Pugnetti L, Caputo D, Cornelio F, Capobianco S, Cesarani A. Vestibular evoked myogenic potentials in multiple sclerosis: clinical and imaging correlations. Mult Scler 2004;10(3):316–321

78. Halmagyi GM, Curthoys IS. A clinical sign of canal paresis. Arch Neurol 1988;45(7):737–739

79. Cremer PD, Halmagyi GM, Aw ST, et al. Semicircular canal plane head impulses detect absent function of individual semicircular canals. Brain 1998;121(Pt 4):699–716

80. Nyström A, Tjernström F, Magnusson M. Outward versus inward head thrusts with video-head impulse testing in normal subjects: does it matter? Otol Neurotol 2015;36(3):e87–e94

81. Halmagyi GM, Weber KP, Aw ST, Todd MJ, Curthoys IS. Impulsive testing of semicircular canal function. Prog Brain Res 2008;171:187–194

82. MacDougall HG, Weber KP, McGarvie LA, Halmagyi GM, Curthoys IS. The video head impulse test: diagnostic accuracy in peripheral vestibulopathy. Neurology 2009;73(14):1134–1141

83. Tian J, Crane BT, Demer JL. Vestibular catch-up saccades in labyrinthine deficiency. Exp Brain Res 2000;131(4):448–457

84. Macdougall HG, Curthoys IS. Plasticity during vestibular compensation: the role of saccades. Front Neurol 2012;3:21

85. Manzari L, Burgess AM, MacDougall HG, Curthoys IS. Vestibular function after vestibular neuritis. Int J Audiol 2013;52(10):713–718

86. Yip CW, Glaser M, Frenzel C, Bayer O, Strupp M. Comparison of the bedside head-impulse test with the video head-impulse test in a clinical practice setting: a prospective study of 500 outpatients. Front Neurol 2016;7:58

87. Black RA, Halmagyi GM, Thurtell MJ, Todd MJ, Curthoys IS. The active head-impulse test in unilateral peripheral vestibulopathy. Arch Neurol 2005;62(2):290–293

88. Kaplan DM, Slovik Y. How do I manage – the head thrust test: technique, usefulness, and limitations. Mediterr J Otol 2005;1:144–147

89. McCaslin DL, Jacobson GP, Bennett ML, Gruenwald JM, Green AP. Predictive properties of the video head impulse test: measures of caloric symmetry and self-report dizziness handicap. Ear Hear 2014;35(5):e185–e191

90. McCaslin DL, Rivas A, Jacobson GP, Bennett ML. The dissociation of video head impulse test (vHIT) and bithermal caloric test results provide topological localization of vestibular system impairment in patients with "definite" Ménière's disease. Am J Audiol 2015;24(1):1–10

91. Curthoys IS, MacDougall HG, McGarvie LA, et al. The video head impulse test. In: Jacobson GP, Shepard NT, eds. Balance Function Assessment and Management. 2nd ed. San Diego, CA: Plural Publishing; 2016:391–430

92. Zellhuber S, Mahringer A, Rambold HA. Relation of video-head-impulse test and caloric irrigation: a study on the recovery in unilateral vestibular neuritis. Eur Arch Otorhinolaryngol 2014;271(9):2375–2383

4 Amplification

● What Type of Evaluation Is Required for Determining Hearing Aid Candidacy?

A **comprehensive audiometric evaluation** is required prior to determining hearing aid candidacy. It is vital that, at a minimum, air and bone conduction (AC and BC) thresholds, speech recognition thresholds (SRT), and word recognition scores (WRSs) be obtained. In addition, tympanometry, acoustic reflex thresholds, and acoustic reflex decay should be performed in patients with asymmetries in audiometric configuration and/or WRSs, conductive or mixed hearing loss, or in patients with subjective reports of pain and/or pressure, dizziness, and/or unilateral tinnitus.

● What Is the Role of the Otologist in Determining Hearing Aid Candidacy?

It is important that the referring physician, preferably an otologist, provide **medical clearance** for amplification prior to a trial period with hearing aids. The U.S. Food and Drug Administration (FDA)[1] requires that medical clearance be obtained for all individuals *under* 18 years. In addition, individuals *over* 18 years should either obtain medical clearance or sign a waiver acknowledging they were informed of the recommendation for medical clearance but elected to proceed with amplification without consulting a physician. It is especially important that patients with asymmetries in audiometric configuration and/or WRSs, conductive or mixed hearing loss, reports of unilateral tinnitus, pain and/or pressure, and dizziness be evaluated by an otologist to determine whether further testing or medical treatment is recommended prior to pursuing amplification. Once medical clearance has been obtained it is safe to proceed with a **hearing aid fitting** (**HAF**). Finally, it is **required** that an audiometric evaluation be completed in 6 months or less before hearing aids are dispensed.

● What Is the Hearing Aid Evaluation?

Typically, a **hearing aid evaluation** (**HAE**) follows the comprehensive evaluation and preferably after medical clearance has been received. The HAE consists of reviewing the results from the audiometric evaluation, counsel on the impact of his/her hearing loss upon communication in quiet, noise, and reverberation, determining patient motivation, and making recommendations for amplification and methods to couple the hearing aids to the patient's ears based on a combination of the patient's hearing loss characteristics, lifestyle, and financial resources.

The HAE begins with a thorough description of the patient's audiometric results to determine hearing aid candidacy and establish realistic expectations with hearing aids in a variety of listening situations and depending upon the patient's hearing loss and ability to recognize speech. For example, a patient with mild–to–moderate sensorineural hearing loss from 2,000 to 8,000 Hz with excellent WRSs is likely to have a better outcome than a patient with severe sensorineural hearing loss and a very poor ability to recognize speech. The use of a **subjective questionnaire** regarding a patient's communication abilities without amplification is also recommended during the HAE. Questionnaires provide the audiologist and patient with a realistic picture of the patient's functional communication abilities in everyday life without amplification and are also used after the HAF to confirm the presence of hearing aid benefit and/or satisfaction. Examples of commonly used questionnaires are the **Abbreviated Profile of Hearing Aid Benefit** (**APHAB**),[2] the **Client Oriented Scale of Improvement** (**COSI**)[3] and the **Characteristics of Amplification Tool** (**COAT**).[4]

● What Are the Available Styles of Hearing Aids?

Once hearing aid candidacy has been determined and the patient feels ready to proceed with amplification, differences in hearing aid styles, levels of technology, and the duration of the repair warranty (1–3 years), as well as loss and damage (1–3 years) are discussed at length.

Hearing aid style refers to the physical appearance of hearing aids and this can be divided into two major categories: custom **in-the-ear** (**ITE; Fig. 4.1a–c**) and behind-the-ear (**BTE**) (**Fig. 4.1d–f**). ITE hearing aids are custom made to each patient's ear(s) and vary in size from an in-the-canal (**ITC; Fig. 4.1a**), **completely-in-the-canal** (**Fig. 4.1b**) and ITE (**Fig. 4.1c**).

With custom hearing aids, all the electronic components are housed in the hearing aid shell that sits in the ear canal and/or part of the concha bowl. Custom hearing aids are typically easier to insert and remove and may have manual controls such as a program button and volume control. Because the electronic components of custom hearing aids are located in a shell that can be deeply inserted in the ear canal, these aids are subject to greater repair due to issues related to cerumen and moisture infiltration into the hearing aids. In addition, the amount of gain available in custom hearing aids is limited due to problems related with feedback (FB).

BTE hearing aids are non-custom and vary in size and the way in which they are coupled to the ear as well as the location of the receiver. **Conventional BTEs** (**Fig. 4.1d**) are coupled to the ear via plastic tubing connected to the earhook of the hearing aid and the tubing and inserted into a custom earmold placed in the ear canal. **Thin-tube receiver-in-the aid** (**RITA**) BTEs (**Fig. 4.1e and again in Fig. 4.2 left**) are be fit with the thin-tube directly connected to the hearing aid and then inserted into a "stock dome" or custom earmold. Finally, **receiver-in-the canal** (**RIC**) BTEs are becoming increasingly popular where the receiver is attached to the hearing aid via a thin wire encased in the plastic tubing (**Fig. 4.1e and again in Fig. 4.2 right**) and then inserted into a "stock dome" or custom earmold. Generally, BTEs are less likely than ITEs to need repairs resulting from moisture and/ or cerumen. In addition, BTEs are usually able to accommodate a wider range of hearing loss (from slight to profound), are less prone to FB-related problems, and have a longer battery life than ITEs.

A derivative of RITA and RICs are **open-fit** hearing aids that are coupled to the ear using a nonoccluding "stock dome" or custom earmold. This fitting option is most appropriate for patients with relatively normal hearing in the low frequencies (250–1,000 Hz) and primarily high-frequency (> 1,000 Hz) hearing loss. When using an open fit, low-frequency sounds enter and exit the open ear canal naturally and amplification is provided only in the middle and/or high frequencies where it is required due to the greater hearing loss in the high frequencies. When the normally open ear canal is completely or partially blocked by an earmold or custom hearing aid, bone-conducted sound is amplified in the space occupying the ear canal from the tip of the earmold/hearing aid to the tympanic membrane by as much as 30 dB in the low frequencies.[5] This phenomenon is known as the **occlusion effect** (**OE**) and results in the patient perceiving that he/she is talking in a barrel which can be very annoying and disruptive. Open-fit hearing aids help to minimize and oftentimes eliminate the OE.

Fig. 4.3 demonstrates a procedure used by audiologists to objectively verify the magnitude of the OE in decibels of **sound pressure level** (**dB SPL**). In this

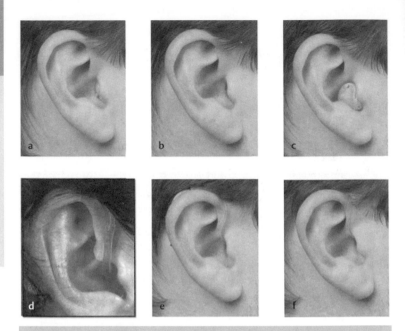

Fig. 4.1 Various styles of hearing aids: (**a**) in-the-canal (ITC), (**b**) completely-in-the-canal (CIC), (**c**) in-the-ear (ITE), (**d**) conventional behind-the-ear (BTE), (**e**) thin-tube receiver in the aid (RITA) BTE, and (**f**) receiver-in-the-canal (RIC) BTE. Photos (**a–c** and **e–f**) are provided courtesy of ReSound Inc.

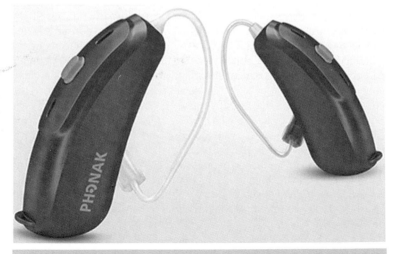

Fig. 4.2 Example of a thin-tube RITA BTE (left) and RIC BTE hearing aid. Photo is provided courtesy of Phonak Inc.

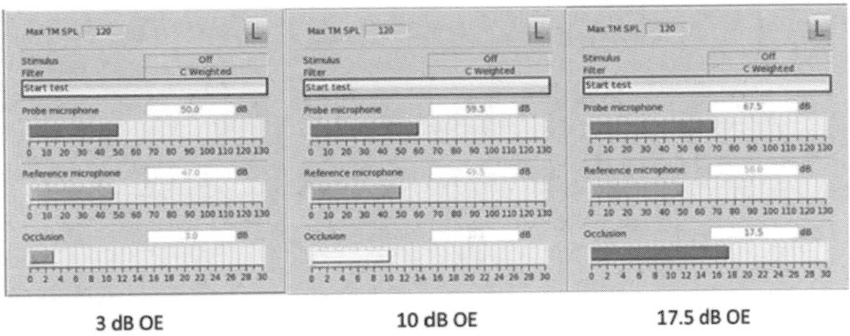

3 dB OE   10 dB OE   17.5 dB OE

Fig. 4.3 Real ear measure of the occlusion effect (OE). Left is an example of minimal OE (3.0 dB), middle is an example of moderate OE (10 dB), and right is an example of severe OE (17.5 dB). Photo is provided courtesy of Etymonic Design Inc.

example, **real ear measures** (REM), which will described in greater detail a later section, is used. In using REM, a **reference microphone** is placed over the ear and a **probe** microphone is placed into the ear canal of the aided ear. The reference microphone is placed outside the ear and is used to measure the input level to the ear. A thin silicone probe tube attached to the probe microphone is inserted into the ear canal so the tip is ~4 to 6 mm from the eardrum. With the hearing aid inserted into the ear, but turned off, the patient is asked to vocalize the vowel "ee" and the amount of intensity present is measured at the reference and probe microphones. As can be seen in **Fig. 4.3**, the dB SPL level measured at the reference microphone and is fairly stable between 47.0 and 50.0 dB SPL for the three measures, but the dB SPL measured by the probe tube varies from 50 to 67.5 dB SPL with the resulting OE between 3.0 and 17.5 dB. An OE of 3 dB is excellent and the patient will not report that he/she feels as if his/her head is in a barrel when speaking. An OE of 17.5 dB, however, would be very annoying. Methods to reduce the OE include widening the vent or ordering a longer bore for the earmold or custom product which is described in the next section.

● What Are the Options for Earmold Style, Tubing, and Venting?

Another aspect of the HAE is to decide how to couple the hearing aids to the patient's ears. This process is completed using either a custom earmold or a "stock dome." **Earmolds** are custom made for a patient's ears and then couple the BTEs to the ears. The style or size of the earmold varies from a **full-shell** earmold that fills the entire concha bowl to a **very open skeleton-type**

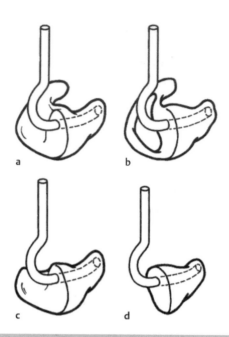

Fig. 4.4 Various earmold styles: (**a**) full shell, (**b**) skeleton, (**c**) half shell, and (**d**) canal. (Reproduced with permission from Microsonic, Inc.)

earmold that is used to secure an open-fit BTE to the ear. Generally, the more severe the hearing loss, the larger the earmold required to provide a better seal allowing for adequate gain without FB. **Fig. 4.4** provides examples of various earmold styles, including a **full-shell, skeleton, half-shell, and canal** earmold.

Plastic **tubing** or a wire encased in a thin-tube in the case of a RIC fitting is necessary to couple the custom earmold to the BTE. The internal diameter, length, and thickness of tubing varies and will change the frequency response generated by the hearing aid which allows for improved customization of the hearing aid to the patient's hearing loss. For example, when an audiologist uses a **Libby Horn** to connect the hearing aid to the earmold, the internal diameter of the tubing increases from 1.93 mm where it connects to the earhook to 3.00 mm at the medial point at the tip of the earmold. This gradual increase in the internal diameter of the tubing provides an enhancement in the high frequencies at 2,800 Hz or greater relative to a tube that maintains the same internal diameter throughout the length of the tubing (i.e., **#13 tubing**). This additional boost in the higher frequencies provided by the Libby Horn has shown to increase speech recognition in quiet and noise relative to using #13 tubing.

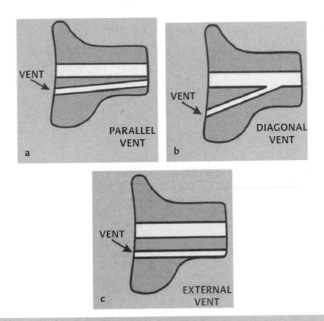

Fig. 4.5. Venting options: (**a**) parallel, (**b**) diagonal (intersecting), and (**c**) trench vent. (Reproduced with permission from Microsonic, Inc. Custom Earmold Manual. 8th ed. Ambridge, PA: Microsonic, Inc.; 2006.)

Venting refers to an open air channel that runs throughout the length of an earmold or hearing aid in the case of an ITE. A vent allows for aeration of the ear canal and provides varying degrees of relief from the OE. Vent types include **parallel, intersecting, and trench**. A parallel vent extends throughout the length of the earmold/custom hearing aid and is parallel to the sound bore; an intersecting vent intersects the sound bore; and a trench vent extends along the entire length of the earmold/custom hearing aid but is drilled on the outside of the earmold/aid. **Fig. 4.5** illustrates the vent types discussed above. The length and diameter of the vent are important in the amount of low- and mid-frequency gain provided by the hearing aid. In general, the more low-frequency gain required, the narrower the vent should be; however, even a patient with a very severe hearing loss should have venting (i.e., **pressure vent**) for comfort and reduction of the OE.

Depending on the style of hearing aids the patient selects an earmold impression is made of each ear canal to order a custom earmold (impressions sent to earmold laboratory) for a BTE impressions for custom ITE hearing aids are sent to the hearing aid manufacturer.

What Are Typical Accessories for Hearing Aids?

Still another component of the HAE is to determine a patient's need or interest in accessories that could be used in combination with his/her hearing aids. Most current hearing aids have **Bluetooth** wireless capability allowing hearing aids to be paired with any number of audio devices (i.e., cell phone, tablet, MP3 player, television, computer, etc.). The most commonly dispensed accessories available from most manufacturers include a remote microphone (**Fig. 4.6a** and **b**), TV listening device (**Fig. 4.6c**), remote control (**Fig. 4.6d**), and remote phone clip (**Fig. 4.6e**).

Remote microphones have been available for years, but until recently, some type of additional **streaming** device was required for the signal from the remote microphone to be received by the hearing aids. The streamer created an additional cost and was felt to be inconvenient, cosmetically unappealing, and therefore often rejected as a viable option. Recently, with the introduction of 2.4 GHz carrier frequency technology, the signal from a remote microphone and other wireless devices can now be directly streamed to the patient's hearing aids. Recent research[6] reported remote microphones can significantly improve the **signal-to-noise ratio** (SNR) for improved performance in a noisy listening environment. In fact, depending upon the listening condition and the make/model of the remote microphone, the improvement in SNR can be as great as 15 to 17 dB. Currently, several remote microphones are available with **automatic adaptive directional** technology so that when placed in a horizontal position (i.e., on a

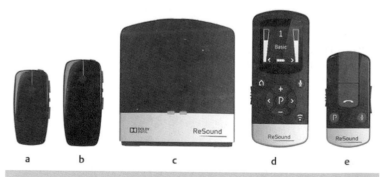

a   b   c   d   e

Fig. 4.6 Several wireless accessories that can be dispensed with hearing aids: (a) remote mini-microphone, (b) remote multi-microphone, (c) TV listening device, (d) remote control, and (e) remote phone clip. Photos are provided courtesy of ReSound Inc.

table) it reverts to an **omnidirectional polar pattern** and provides best performance for listening in quiet environment. When placed in a vertical position (i.e., hanging on a collar or blouse), it reverts to a **hypercardioid directional polar pattern** that provides best performance when listening in a noisy environment.

Another component of the HAE is discussing **smartphone applications** recently made available from several hearing aid manufacturers. Depending on the specific smartphone application, the patient can use his/her cell phone to (1) increase/decrease the volume in one or both hearing aids; (2) change programs that have been programmed into the hearing aids (i.e., meetings, restaurant, telephone, music, car, etc.); (3) stream a remote microphone to his/her hearing aids; (4) find lost hearing aids; (5) fine-tune his/her hearing aids in real time in specific listening environments and then save those responses as a separate programs so when the patient returns to that listening environment the hearing aids automatically retrieve the saved programs via the GPS capability of the cell phone; (6) answer and reject phone calls with the call delivered directly to both of his/her hearing aids.

● What Is the Basic Sound Processing of a Hearing Aid?

Current hearing aids consist of some of the most advanced digital signal processing available; however, the basic sound processing of a hearing aid remains the same today as it did in the past. All hearing aids, analog or digital, consist of a few basic components allowing for sound processing to occur: a **microphone** (or microphones), an **amplifier**, and **receiver** (or loudspeaker). The microphone converts acoustic energy to electric energy, the amplifier amplifies the electronic signal, and the receiver converts the electronic signal back to an acoustic signal. In a digital hearing aid, sound is picked up by one or more microphones and the sound signal is filtered through an analog-to-digital converter. From there, the binary code is sent through an amplifier, where multiple stages of sound processing occur, and then through a digital-to-analog converter. Finally, the amplified sound is delivered to the patient's ear canal via the receiver or loudspeaker. **Fig. 4.7** depicts the basic sound processing discussed above. The advanced sound processing that occurs in the amplification stage, including noise reduction (NR) and FB management, is discussed in the following sections.

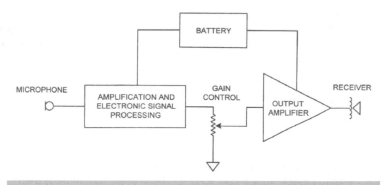

Fig. 4.7 Block diagram depicting the basic sound processing in a hearing aid. (Reproduced with permission from Agnew, J. Amplifiers and circuit algorithms for contemporary hearing aids. In: Valente M, ed. Hearing Aids: Standards, Options, and Limitations. 2nd ed. New York, NY: Thieme Medical Publishers, Inc.;2002:101–142.)

● What Are Directional Microphones and How Do They Work?

The primary complaint of patients with hearing loss is increased difficulty understanding speech in background noise. Oftentimes, patients report that *without* hearing aids (i.e., **unaided**) they do well in quiet listening situations but cannot understand speech when noise is present. Also, in the past, patients *with* hearing aids (i.e., **aided**) reported they did well with their hearing aids in quiet but not nearly as well in noise. That is, aided performance was not significantly better than unaided in noisy listening situations. To address this problem, hearing aids were developed with two or more microphones (i.e., **directional microphone**) to help address this complaint by reducing the level of noise from behind and/or sides of the listener, thereby providing the greatest amplification for sounds arriving from the front. In this way, the hearing aids attempt to make speech more audible in the presence of background noise. Such a system, referred to as a **directional microphone**, improves the SNR. When a hearing aid is only equipped with one microphone or when only the front microphone of a directional microphone system is activated (referred to as **omnidirectional**), then the microphone is equally sensitive to sounds all around the listener. At this point, it must be emphasized that as good as a directional microphone can be in improving the SNR relative to an omni-directional microphone, its performance cannot match the very significant improvement provided by a remote microphone described earlier.

Directional microphones have different **polar patterns** that are measured and described as **polar plots** based on the azimuth(s) at which the microphone provides the least (null) amount of amplification. Also, within each polar plot, each of the six circles represents 5 dB of attenuation. **Fig. 4.8** illustrates a variety of polar plots, including **cardioid**, **bidirectional**, **hypercardioid, and supercardioid**. For example, a directional microphone system with a bidirectional polar pattern (**Fig. 4.8b**) provides the greatest amplification to the front and back of the listener (i.e., because the frequency response is at the first circle) and minimal amplification for sounds arriving directly to the sides (at 90 and 270 degrees azimuth; ~25 dB attenuation because the response it at the sixth inner circle).

The earliest directional microphone systems required the patient to manually select, via a switch on the hearing aids or a remote control, whether the hearing aid would function in omnidirectional or directional mode. The patient was counseled to leave the hearing aid in omnidirectional mode for quiet listening and switch to the directional mode in noisy situations. In addition, the first directional microphone systems were available with one

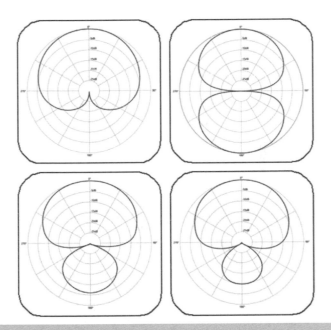

Fig. 4.8. Polar plots for directional microphones: cardioid (**a**), bidirectional (**b**), hypercardioid (**c**), and supercardioid (**d**). (Vector graphics created by user Galak76 for Wikipedia Commons. Permission to reproduce the images is provided under the Creative Commons license. These images appear in their original context under the heading Microphone Polar Patterns on Wikipedia: Microphone. http://en.wikipedia.org/wiki/Microphone. Accessed December 7, 2016.)

fixed polar pattern. With advanced technology, directional microphones are now **automatic and adaptive**. This means that if the signal processing detects that the listening environment is absent of significant noise it will automatically activate only the forward facing microphone and the polar pattern changes to a omnidirectional polar pattern (i.e., no attenuation regardless the azimuth of the signal). Now, if the signal processing detects a sufficient level of noise, the signal processing will automatically activate the back microphone and the polar pattern will automatically adapt and change based on the location and characteristics of the noise.

In addition, current hearing aids vary in the number of **frequency channels** available. Some current commercial hearing aids have as many as **24 channels** (or more) of signal processing. Each frequency channel in a hearing aid is assigned a specified bandwidth that controls the hearing aid compression characteristics (compression allows all sounds to fit into a user's dynamic range so it squeezes or compresses the speech signal so all sounds can be heard), NR, FB management, and directional microphone characteristics. It is helpful to think of channels as keys on a piano or sliders on an audio equalizer board. Importantly, many current digital hearing aids with multiple channels of signal processing perform better in background noise because the polar pattern may vary in each channel and will continually change within each channel based on the input level and characteristics of the incoming noise. Such a directional microphone system is referred to as having **automatic adaptive multichannel directionality** and is the most advanced directional microphone system currently available.

Finally, current digital hearing aids incorporate **"scene analysis."** That is, a variety of typical environmental "scenes" (e.g., quiet listening, restaurant, traffic noise, wind, party, music, TV, etc.) have been analyzed by acoustical engineers from the various hearing aid manufacturers. These "scenes" are then embedded in digital chip of the hearing aid so that when the listener is listening in that "scene," the signal processor automatically manipulates the numerous parameters of the hearing aid (i.e., gain, output, compression kneepoint, compression ratio, NR, directionality, etc.) that would theoretically provide the optimal performance in that "scene." This feature adds to the **automatic signal processing** completed by current digital hearing aids. More expensive hearing aids contain more "scenes." Less expensive hearing aids contain fewer "scenes."

● What Is Noise Reduction?

Hearing aids are constantly analyzing the patient's listening environment in an attempt to provide the best amplification for speech. Speech is a modulated signal that is constantly varying in intensity and frequency, whereas noise is typically a steady-state, broadband signal (e.g., restaurant noise) with greater emphasis in the low-frequency region, or a very sudden and brief increase in intensity (e.g., a door slamming). If hearing aids detect a steady-state signal, or what it believes to be impact noise, the hearing aid will decrease the gain at the frequency region(s) contained in the noise. Most digital hearing aids today provide some type of **noise reduction**; however, the ability of the hearing aid to reduce noise while maintaining the available gain for speech varies greatly depending on the technology employed in each hearing aid. Unlike directional microphones, NR *does not* improve the SNR (i.e., NR reduces both the level of the signal and noise). *NR simply improves comfort in noise by reducing the gain of the hearing aid for noisy situations.*

Fig. 4.9 demonstrates a procedure used to objectively verify the magnitude of NR provided by the hearing aid in dB SPL. In this situation, coupler measures, which will described in greater detail a later section, are used. In using coupler measures, the hearing aid is coupled to a 2-mL coupler and placed in a hearing aid test box. Various types of noise (e.g., air conditioner, multitalker babble) can be presented at various input levels via the software, and the test reports the reduction in the output of the hearing aid as a result of the presence of the specific noise and the specific input level. In **Fig. 4.9**, the

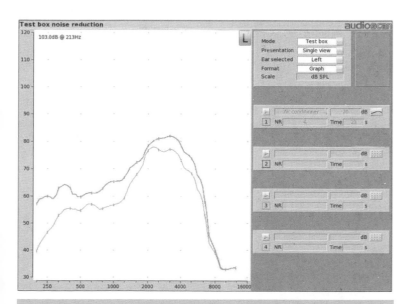

Fig. 4.9 Coupler measure verifying the effectiveness of noise reduction (NR) programmed into a hearing aids. The lower thin line represents the reduction in output (4 dB) as a result of NR.

thinner line reports the amount of reduction of the amplification provided by the NR feature. **Fig. 4.9** reports that overall NR is 4 dB in response to the introduction of the air conditioner noise presented at 70 dB SPL. Again, it is important to emphasize that **NR does not improve speech recognition in noise. NR simply acts to make listening in noisy listening situations less annoying**.

● What Is Feedback Management?

Feedback (**FB**), or the annoying whistle produced by hearing aids, occurs when amplified sound exiting the receiver is reamplified by the hearing aid when it reenters the microphone. Common causes of FB include a poor fitting custom hearing aid or earmold, cerumen in the hearing aid/earmold or in the ear canal, crack in the tubing, or a mechanical problem. A few methods for reducing FB include plugging or narrowing the vent, making a tighter fitting earmold/hearing aid, reducing the gain via the programming software, or reducing the gain manually via the volume control are often effective. If, however, the gain of the hearing aid is reduced, the listener will sacrifice audibility. Most current digital hearing aids incorporate **feedback cancellation** software that virtually eliminates FB before it is audible to the user or communication partner. The majority of FB cancellation systems work by detecting FB and generating a signal of equal frequency and intensity of the FB but of inverse phase to cancel the FB. The major benefit of this FB reduction technology is that the amount of usable gain available to the user is not sacrificed to the degree that it had been in the past. This especially holds true for hearing aids with multiple channels of signal processing, as was discussed in the directional microphone section above, as audibility of sounds in frequency channels where the FB does not exist is completely maintained.

● Which Is Best: Monaural or Bilateral Amplification?

For patients with bilateral symmetrical hearing loss and similar WRSs, bilateral amplification is highly recommended. Input to two ears allows for improved **localization**, **binaural summation**, and **binaural squelch**, as was discussed in Chapter 1. When a listener has the use of only one ear or when one ear is significantly better than the other, the listener's ability to make use of **localization** cues is significantly reduced. In addition, monaural listening requires a greater SNR to communicate effectively because the advantages of binaural summation and squelch are unavailable. **Binaural summation** refers to the perceived loudness increase when listening to a sound with both ears (of approximately equal hearing sensitivity) versus with only one ear. When the intensity of a sound is near the listener's auditory threshold (0 dB **sensation level or SL**) the binaural advantage is ~3 dB, whereas for sounds greater than or equal to 35 dB above threshold (35 dB SL), the binaural advantage is ~6 dB.[7] As a result, patients with bilateral amplification have improved audibility with less gain, which results in less acoustic FB and greater reserve gain in the hearing aids.

Binaural squelch refers to a listener's ability to listen only to the sound source of interest when additional sound sources are present. Hearing in background noise is difficult for both normal-hearing and hearing-impaired listeners, and difficulty hearing in background noise is one of the most common complaints among hearing aid users. As a result, it is recommended that individuals with bilateral hearing loss pursue bilateral amplification to take advantage of binaural squelch. Occasionally, a patient with bilateral hearing loss and asymmetrical word recognition abilities will receive greatest benefit from a monaural HAF in the ear with the better WRS; however, because it is difficult to predict which individuals will benefit most from a monaural fitting, it is best practice to recommend a trial period with bilateral amplification. During the trial period, the patient can experiment with using one or both hearing aids to determine if bilateral amplification or monaural amplification is preferred. In the author's experience, when using this strategy ~85% of patients prefer bilateral amplification, whereas ~15% prefer monaural amplification.

● What Are Available Hearing Aid Options for Unilateral Hearing Loss?

Several hearing aid options are available for patients with **unilateral hearing loss**, which is sometimes referred to as **single-sided deafness (SSD)**. These options include **bone-anchored hearing aid** (**BAHA; Fig. 4.10a**), **TransEar (Fig. 4.10b)**, and wireless **contralateral routing of the signal** (**CROS; Fig. 4.10c**).

In the case of SSD, the BAHA is a device that is coupled to a surgically implanted titanium screw and abutment in the mastoid bone of the "dead" ear and uses BC to transmit sounds from the ear with hearing loss to the ear with normal BC thresholds of 20 dB HL or less from 500 to 3,000 Hz. More current BAHAs can be coupled to the mastoid via a magnet. The BAHA can

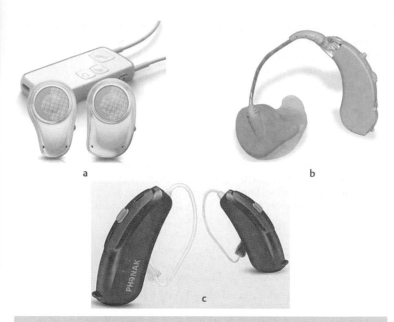

Fig. 4.10 Three device options for unilateral hearing loss: (**a**) BAHA, (**b**) TransEar bone-conduction hearing aid, and (**c**) wireless CROS system consisting of an FM transmitter and receiver. Photo **a** is provided courtesy of Oticon Medical. Photo **b** is provided courtesy of EarTech Inc. Photo **c** is provided courtesy of Phonak Inc.

also be used on patients with **conductive** and **mixed** hearing loss. Also, as seen in **Fig. 4.10a**, current BAHAs use wireless connectivity. The rectangular object in the upper portion of **Fig. 4.10a** is a streamer allowing the user to wirelessly communicate with his/her cell phone, control volume, and change programs. The streamer can also interact with other wireless devices allowing for wireless streaming of a phone, TV, and remote microphone. Finally, as with hearing aids, the BAHA can also communicate with smartphone apps.

TransEar (Ear Technology Corp., Johnson City, TN) is a BTE digital hearing aid that connects via a wire to a tightly fit custom ITC shell with a long bore length so the tip rests on the bony portion of the ear canal. The custom shell houses a small BC vibrator, allowing sounds stimulating the poor ear to be transmitted to the inner ear of the good ear via BC.

A wireless CROS involves the use of a frequency modulated (FM) transmitting microphone on the poor ear (**left hearing aid in Fig. 4.10c**) that sends sound from the poor ear to an FM receiver in the good ear (**right hearing aid in Fig. 4.10c**) via an open earmold.

FDA guidelines recommend that the BC pure-tone average (500–3,000 Hz) in the normal ear be 20 dB HL or better for greatest success with BAHA fittings for SSD. No such FDA guideline exists for TransEar or CROS options discussed above; however, logic would suggest that the guideline of BC thresholds of 20 dB HL or better be used for the TransEar because the mode of transmission (BC) is similar for each.

Recently the use of a **cochlear implant** (**CI**) implanted into the poor ear for patients with SSD has increased. In some recent reports, it has been found that the CI can possibly provide improved localization to patients with SSD which has not been an outcome with any other treatment option for SSD. Currently, the CI has not been approved by the FDA for SSD, but it is very possible that the FDA will approve this application in the near future.

● What Are Coupler Measurements and Why Are They Important?

It is impossible to confirm that a hearing aid is working properly simply by listening to it. As a result, it is imperative that **electroacoustic measurements** be performed to ensure that the hearing aids (*new and repaired*) meet technical specifications (ANSI S3.22–2009[8]). Such measurements are performed in a standardized test chamber upon receipt of a new *and* repaired hearing aid and at each hearing aid check appointment. Hearing aid test systems consist of a sound chamber that includes one or more **loudspeaker(s)** (i.e., large circular component in the back of **Fig. 4.11a–c**). As an additional note, the manufacturer of the analyzer illustrated in **Fig. 4.11a–c** also has two additional loudspeakers embedded in the lid closing the test chamber. These loudspeakers generate standardized test signals (pure-tones, speech-weighted signals, actual speech), various **hearing aid couplers** (e.g., circular components in **Fig. 4.11a–c** in which the hearing aid is attached), a **reference microphone** (e.g., long stick-like component in **Fig. 4.11a–c**) that is placed at the input to the microphone of the hearing aid and used to control the input level (in dB SPL) to the microphone of the hearing aid. The coupler approximates the volume of the average adult ear canal (2 mL), and a measuring microphone is placed inside the coupler to send the amplified signal to an analyzer to record the response of the hearing aid to the various input signals. **Fig. 4.11** demonstrates a BTE (a), RIC (b), and ITE (c) hearing aid attached to 2-mL couplers in the test box for electroacoustic assessment.

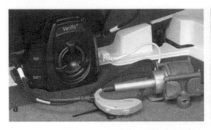
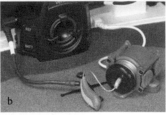
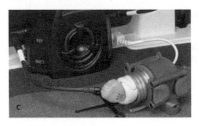

Fig. 4.11 (**a**) BTE attached to an HA-2, 2-mL coupler; (**b**) RIC BTE attached to an HA-1, 2-mL coupler; and (**c**) ITE attached to an HA-1, 2-mL coupler for electro-acoustic assessment. Photo is provided courtesy of Etymonic Inc.

Two commonly performed coupler measurements are **ANSI S3.22–2009**[8] and **S3.42–1992**.[9] Electroacoustic analysis using ANSI S3.42–1992 is useful to determine if a hearing aid has linear or nonlinear signal processing and if excessive **intermodulation distortion (IMD)** is present. **Fig. 4.12** illustrates a family of frequency response curves to input levels of pink noise presented at 50, 60, 70, and 80 dB SPL. As is illustrated in **Fig. 4.12**, the output of frequency response curves increase in equal amounts as the input signal is increased in 10 dB steps, which is indicative of linear signal processing.

Another potential use of ANSI S3.42–1992 is to determine if the hearing aid has excessive IMD. It can be seen in **Fig. 4.12**, the morphology, or shape of the frequency response curve for the 80 dB SPL input, although showing more output, has the same shape as the frequency response curve for the 50 dB SPL input signal. If this hearing aid had excessive IMD, the frequency response for the higher input level would appear "jagged" or "broken-up." In that case, it would be best practice to attach the printout to the manufacturer repair form and explain that the attached measure suggests the presence of IMD and the hearing aid needs to be repaired. Excessive IMD can result in poor sound quality and reduced ability to understand speech in quiet and noisy listening environments.

ANSI S3.22–2009 (**Fig. 4.13**) is a standardized test that uses a swept (200–8,000 Hz) pure-tone signal to measure the performance of the hearing aid relative to the manufacturer specification. The measured values obtained during an ANSI S3.22–2009 measurement include the maximum output (108 dB SPL), average output (97 dB SPL), output SPL curve using a 90 dB SPL pure-tone sweep (upper green curve), frequency response curve (lower red curve), frequency range (450–6,300 Hz), average gain (17 dB at input levels of 50 and 60 dB SPL), equivalent input noise level (44 dB SPL), total harmonic distortion (2% at 500, 1% at 800 Hz and 0% at 1,600 Hz), telecoil response (not reported in **Fig. 4.13**), battery drain (not reported in **Fig. 4.13**), and the compression characteristics of a hearing aid (not reported in **Fig. 4.13**). After completing electroacoustic assessment, the response of a hearing aid should be compared with manufacturer's specification to ensure that the patient is receiving a quality product that is functioning properly. This measurement is required for *new* and *repaired* hearing aids and should become a part of the patient's medical record. This test can also be completed at scheduled semi-annual or annual patient visits, unscheduled patient visits where the patient has a specific complaint about the performance of the hearing aid(s), and at the HAF following programming.

Another important coupler measure to perform when new hearing aids arrive is to verify that the directional microphone is attenuating signals arriving from the sides or back (i.e., the frequency response of

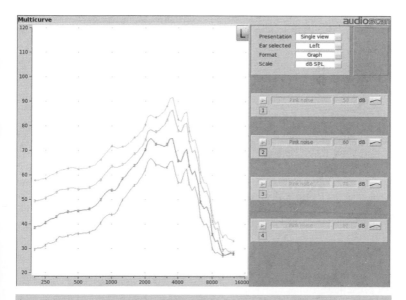

Fig. 4.12 Example of a 2-mL coupler measurement of a digital BTE hearing aid using multicurve program in hearing aid test box. In this example, the output of the hearing aid is measured for pink noise at input levels 50, 60, 70, and 80 dB SPL.

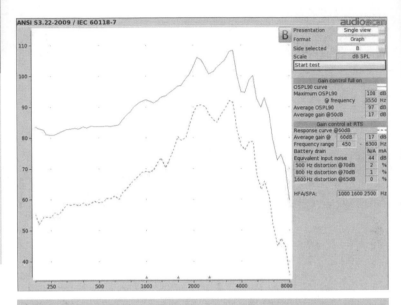

Fig. 4.13 Example of a 2-mL coupler measurement of a BTE to ANSI S3.22–2009.

the hearing aid in response to signals arriving from the back is reduced [attenuated] relative to the frequency response of the hearing aid in response to signals arriving from the front). On occasion, new hearing aids will arrive where the directional microphone is not operating at all. That is, when assessing the coupler performance of the directional microphone it is seen that the hearing aid is operating as an omnidirectional microphone (i.e., the frequency response of the hearing aid in response to signals arriving from the front and back loudspeakers are superimposed). Also, it is possible that new hearing aids will be shipped where the directional microphones is reversed. That is, sounds arriving from behind are amplified, whereas sounds arriving from the front are attenuated. Clearly, this is not desirable and this aid would need to be returned to the manufacturer to be replaced by a new hearing aid.

Fig. 4.14 demonstrates a procedure used to objectively verify the magnitude of the attenuation provided by a directional microphone. In this situation, coupler measures are used. In using coupler measures, the hearing aid is coupled to a 2-mL coupler and placed in a hearing aid test box. Signals are presented from a forward and rear facing loudspeaker. Various types of signals can be introduced via the test box. In **Fig. 4.14**, the upper bold green curve represents the frequency response to the forward facing loudspeaker, whereas the thinner lower green curve represents the frequency response

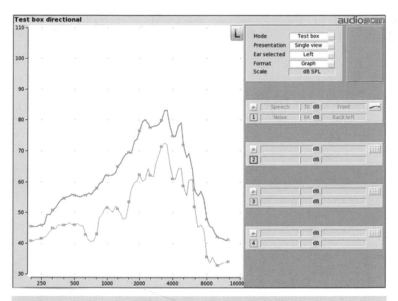

Fig. 4.14 Example of a coupler front-to-back measure of a hearing aid with a directional microphone. The upper curve is the response of the hearing aid to the front loudspeaker, and the lower curve is the response of the hearing aid to the rear facing loudspeaker. The difference between these two curves is the magnitude of noise reduction provided by the directional microphone with sounds arriving from behind.

of the hearing aid to the rear facing loudspeaker. As can be seen, there is a significant reduction in the output of the hearing aid when the signal is presented to the hearing aid from the rear facing microphone.

● What Are Prescriptive Targets and How Are They Used?

The amount of gain or output prescribed for hearing aids at each frequency cannot be arbitrarily derived. Much like a vision examination results in a prescription for glasses or contact lenses, each patient's audiometric thresholds are used to prescribe the appropriate amount of gain or output at 200 to 8,000 Hz to allow soft speech (50 dB SPL) to be audible and judged as sounding "soft"; average speech (60–65 dB SPL) to be intelligible and judged as sounding "comfortably loud," and loud speech (80 dB SPL) to be "loud, but OK." Though several prescriptive methods exist, the two most commonly used by audiologists are **NAL-NL2**[10] and **DSL v5.0**.[11] NAL-NL2, the **National**

Acoustic Laboratories (**NAL**) fitting strategy for linear and nonlinear signal processing, attempts to maximize speech intelligibility while equalizing loudness. The **DSL v5.0** method, which stands for **Desired Sensation Level** (**DSL**), was originally developed for determining the prescribed hearing aid gain or output for children and attempts to normalize loudness. **Real ear verification** measures, which are discussed in detail in the next section, are performed to confirm that the measured gain or output of a hearing aid is meeting the prescriptive target for the patient's hearing loss.

Fig. 4.15 reports **REM** for a hearing aid programmed to NAL-NL2. The upper *black asterisks* represent the *prescribed* maximum output using a 90 dB SPL input from 250 to 8,000 Hz for the hearing aid based on the audiometric thresholds of the patient. The *yellow* curve is the *measured* output using a 90 dB SPL sweep. It can be seen that the *measured programmed* output is

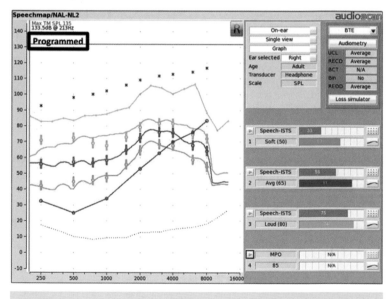

Fig. 4.15 Real ear aided response (REAR) measurement for a hearing aid programmed to NAL-NL2 for input levels of 50, 65, and 80 dB SPL. Curve 1 (green) = output of hearing aid to a soft input (50 dB SPL), curve 2 (pink) = output of hearing aid to an average input (65 dB SPL), curve 3 (blue) = output of the hearing aid to a loud input level (80 dB SPL), and curve 4 (yellow) = maximum output of the hearing aid in response to a 90 dB SPL signal. This is a well-fit hearing aid, as the output for each input level very closely approximates the prescribed targets for soft (green symbol), average (pink symbols), and loud (blue symbols), and the maximum output of the hearing aid (yellow curve) does not exceed the patient's predicted maximum loudness discomfort level (black asterisks).

below the *prescribed* maximum output and therefore loud sounds should not be judged to be uncomfortably loud. The *blue symbols* represent the *prescribed* output for an 80 dB SPL input level, and the *blue curve* represents the *measured programmed* output to the same signal. It can be seen that the measured response closely matches the prescribed curve. The *red symbols* represent the *prescribed* output for a 65 dB SPL input level, and the *red curve* represents the *measured programmed* output to the same signal. It can be seen that the *measured* response closely matches the *prescribed* curve. The *green symbols* represent the *prescribed* output for a 50 dB SPL input level, and the *green curve* represents the *measured programmed* output to the same signal. Again, it can be seen that the *measured programmed* response closely matches the prescribed curve. Finally, the lower solid **red** curve represents the patient's audiometric threshold measured in dB HL converted to dB SPL measured near the eardrum, and the lower thin black curve represents the threshold of normal listeners converted to dB SPL measured near the eardrum. The area between the patient's threshold (red curve) and maximum output (black asterisk) represents the patient's **dynamic range**, and the goal of the fitting is to be sure the measured output for soft (50 dB SPL), average (65 dB SPL), and loud (80 dB SPL) speech fits within the dynamic range of the patient and that a loud input level (90 dB SPL) does not exceed the prescribed maximum output.

The lower curves in **Fig. 4.16** is the prescribed and programmed **Real Ear Insertion Gain** (**REIG**) for a hearing aid using 50 (green), 65 (red), and 80 (blue) dB SPL of pink noise. Again, notice how close the measured responses match the prescribed responses.

● What Are Real Ear Measurements and Why Are They Important?

Two national **Best Practice Guidelines**[12,13] suggest that REM should be performed on *all* HAFs to verify that the gain or output provided by the hearing aids to a patient matches, as closely as possible, a valid prescribed target that was described in the previous section (e.g., **Figs. 4.15** and **4.16**) Unfortunately, ~75 to 80% of audiologists fail to perform REMs regularly.[14] As a result, many hearing aid users achieve inadequate amplification, especially in the higher frequencies (**Fig. 4.17**), which decreases overall speech intelligibility and hearing aid satisfaction. In **Fig. 4.17**, notice how the measured responses for 50, 65, and 80 dB SPL fall significantly fall below the prescribed targets (i.e., under amplifying).

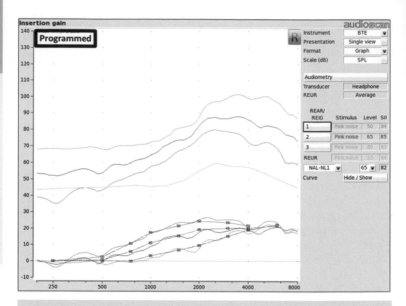

Fig. 4.16 Real ear insertion gain (REIG) measurement for an input level of 50 dB SPL (upper green curve), 65 dB SPL (middle pink curve), and 80 dB SPL (blue curve). This is a well-fit hearing aid, as the gain for each input level very closely approximates the prescribed targets(dotted lines) for soft (green curve), average (pink curve), and loud (blue curve).

Much like coupler measurements verify that hearing aids meet ANSI specifications, **REM** verify that a hearing aid is appropriately amplifying sound in a patient's ear canal. Each hearing aid manufacturer provides software that contains a manufacturer proprietary **"first-fit"** (**Fig. 4.17**) algorithm that calculates the gain or output required to meet their target based on a patient's hearing loss. Hearing aid manufacturers, however, use *average* data to determine the maximum output, gain and output characteristics of hearing aids, and as a result, the "first-fit" prescribed by a manufacturer almost always results in hearing aids being fit inappropriately (i.e., inadequate high-frequency gain or output). In addition, the size and shape of an individual ear canal have unique resonant properties, which greatly influence the way that the sound exiting the hearing aid receiver is actually amplified. As a result, it is imperative that REM be performed at the initial HAF *for all hearing aids* to ensure that soft sounds (i.e., 50 dB SPL) are "soft," but audible, that input levels approximating average speech (i.e., 60–65 dB SPL) are "'comfortably loud," and that loud sounds (i.e., 80 dB SPL) are "loud, but OK."

REM uses a very thin silicone probe tube that is attached to a probe microphone that is inserted into the ear canal so the tip is ~4 to 6 mm from the

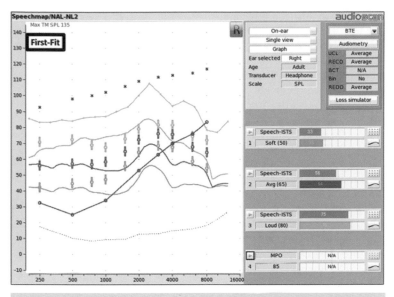

Fig. 4.17 Real ear aided response (REAR) measurement for a hearing aid programmed to NAL-NL2 for input levels of 50, 65, and 80 dB SPL **using manufacturer first-fit**. Note that in each input level the measured response does not match the NAL-NL2 target.

tympanic membrane to measure the level of unamplified and amplified sound (dB SPL). REM verifies that soft (50 dB SPL), average (65 dB SPL), and loud (80 dB SPL) levels of speech are amplified appropriately by comparing the measured gain or output of the hearing aid to the prescriptive target for each input level for the patient's hearing loss. Patient configuration for REMs consists of a loudspeaker located ~12 in from the test ear(s), a reference microphone located at ear level that confirms the level of sound reaching the ear from the loudspeaker is accurate, and a probe tube from a probe microphone placed in the ear canal so the tip of the probe tube is ~4 to 6 mm from the tympanic membrane.

The most commonly performed real ear tests are **REIG** (**Fig. 4.16**) and **Real Ear Aided Response** (**REAR; Figs. 4.15** and **4.17**) measurements. REIG measures the gain provided by the hearing aids, whereas REAR measures the output provided by the hearing aids. REIG measurements subtract the ear canal resonance, referred to as **Real Ear Unaided Gain** (**REUG**), from the **Real Ear Aided Gain** (**REAG**) of the hearing aid. Therefore, REIG = REAG − REUG. **Fig. 4.16** illustrates REIG measurements. REAR measures the output (i.e., input level + the gain provided by the hearing aids) of the hearing aid in dB SPL;

therefore, an unaided measurement of the ear canal resonance is not required. **Fig. 4.15** illustrates real ear SPL measurements on what is commonly referred to as an **SPL-O-Gram**. As the audiologist performs REM at each input level (50, 65, and 80 dB SPL), fine-tuning adjustments are made to the hearing aid(s) via the manufacturer software to be sure the measured gain or output more closely approximates the prescriptive target. In addition, REM confirms that the maximum output of the hearing aid never exceeds a patient's LDLs. This is confirmed by comparing the response of the hearing aid to a 90 dB SPL pure-tone sweep, referred to as the **Real Ear Saturation Response** (**RESR90**), to the patient's LDLs. In addition, subjective aided loudness judgments for *speech* presented at 50, 65, and 80 dB SPL should be recorded where the patient reports how loud the speech signal is on a scale from 1 to 7 where 1 is a rating of "very soft" and 7 is a rating of "uncomfortably loud." In a patient with well-fit hearing aid(s), a speech signal at 50 dB SPL should be rated from 1 to 3, at 65 dB SPL it should be rated from 3 to 5, and at 80 dB SPL it should be rated at less than 7.

● What Is the Difference between Verification and Validation?

The **verification** of hearing aids (coupler, real ear, aided sound-field thresholds, aided WRSs in quiet and noise) is an objective measurement of hearing aid performance, whereas **validation** refers to a subjective assessment of hearing aid benefit/performance. Verification occurs via the use of specialized equipment to confirm that hearing aids are providing adequate gain for soft, average, and loud inputs, and that loud sounds are never uncomfortably loud. Validation employs the use of subjective questionnaires, such as the APHAB,[2] COSI,[3] and COAT,[4] to determine if the hearing aids are meeting the needs of the patient, according to the patient. Both measures are important in determining the success of an HAF and should be employed for all HAFs to provide the highest level of quality patient care and to determine the need for further hearing aid programming, counseling, and/or aural rehabilitation to provide patients with the greatest possible benefits from their hearing aids.

● What Is Hearing Assistance Technology?

Hearing Assistance Technology (**HAT**) is any device, other than a hearing aid, that is used to enhance communication in everyday life. Devices such as remote microphones, amplified telephones, TV listening devices, amplified stethoscopes, alerting systems, and personal FM, radio frequency (RF), or infrared listening systems are a few examples of HAT (**Fig. 4.18**). Such devices may be used in conjunction with or independent of hearing aids. For patients with difficulty in word recognition abilities, HAT is often a requirement for successful communication in adverse listening situations because the use of HAT increases the SNR and overcomes the adverse factors such as background noise, distance, and reverberation.

When HAT devices are used in conjunction with hearing aids, the hearing aids may require either a telecoil or an FM receiver to pick up the signal of interest. For example, a personal FM system consists of an external microphone (transmitter) and an FM receiver. The transmitter is worn within 6 to 12 in of the communication partner's mouth, and the signal that is picked up by the transmitter microphone is delivered via an FM signal (also referred to as RF signal) to the patient's hearing aid. The patient's hearing aid must have either an FM receiver attached to it or the patient must have an active telecoil in the hearing aid, which is a small copper coil that receives

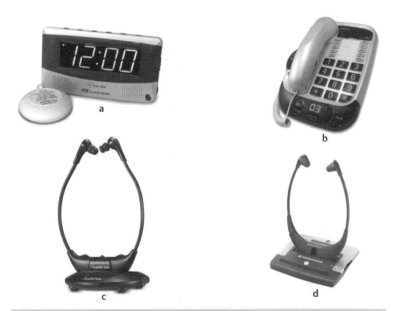

Fig. 4.18 Various HAT devices: (**a**) travel alarm clock with FM radio and vibrating bed shaker, (**b**) digital amplified speaker phone, (**c**) wireless **radio frequency** TV listening device with a 2.4 GHz frequency transmission, and (**d**) wireless **infrared** TV listening device with a 2.3 MHz frequency transmission. Photos are provided courtesy of Oaktree Products.

an audio signal via magnetic leakage from a loop worn around the patient's neck. While an FM transmission is very clear and allows the listener to be within 75 ft from the transmitter, other HAT devices deliver the signal of interest to the patient's ears via an infrared transmission, which requires direct line-of-sight to function properly and may be interrupted if the line-of-sight is compromised by sunlight or some physical barrier. Many television listening devices use an infrared transmission, much like a television remote.

Finally, telephone use is often difficult for individuals with hearing loss. Amplified telephones, captioned telephones, and TTY/TDD (teletypewriter/ telecommunications device for the deaf) devices are options for patients with varying degrees of hearing loss and aural/oral communication abilities. Other HAT devices exist to improve the quality of life of individuals with hearing impairment. Such devices include alarm clocks, doorbell systems, smoke detectors, and wrist watches with alarm vibration and amplification, flashing lights, and/or vibration that are used to alert the hearing impaired listener.

References

1. U.S. Food and Drug Administration. Code of Federal Regulations, Title 21: Food and Drugs. (Revised April 1, 2007). 21CFR801.421. Washington, DC: Government Printing Office
2. Cox RM, Alexander GC. The abbreviated profile of hearing aid benefit. Ear Hear 1995;16(2):176–186
3. Dillon H, James A, Ginis J. Client oriented scale of improvement (COSI) and its relationship to several other measures of benefit and satisfaction provided by hearing aids. J Am Acad Audiol 1997;8(1):27–43
4. Sandridge SA, Newman CW. Improving the efficiency and accountability of the hearing aid selection process—use of the COAT. http://www.audiologyonline.com/articles/article_detail.asp?article_ id=1541. Accessed April 20, 2009
5. Revit LJ. Two techniques for dealing with the occlusion effect. Hear Instrum 1992;43(12):16–18
6. Rodemerk KS, Galster JA. Benefits of remote microphones using four wireless protocols. J Am Acad Audiol 2015;26(8):724–731
7. Gelfand SA. Hearing: An Introduction to Psychological and Physiological Acoustics. 4th ed. New York, NY: Marcel Dekker; 2004
8. American National Standards Institute. American National Standard for Specification of Hearing Aid Characteristics (ANSI S3.22–2009). New York, NY: ANSI

9.   American National Standards Institute. American National Standard for Testing Hearing Aids with a Broad-Band Noise Signal. (ANSI S3.42–1992). New York, NY: ANSI

10.   Keidser G, Dillon H, Flax M, Ching T, Brewer S. The NAL-NL2 prescriptive procedure. Audiol Res 2011;1:88–90

11.   Scollie S, Seewald R, Cornelisse L, et al. The Desired sensation level multistage input/output algorithm. Trends Amplif 2005;9(4):159–197

12.   ASHA Ad Hoc Committee on Hearing Aid Selection and Fitting. Guidelines for hearing aid fitting for adults. Am J Audiol 1998;7(1):5–13

13.   Valente M. Guidelines for the audiological management of adult hearing impairment. Audiol Today 2006;18(5):32–36

14.   Mueller G, Picou E. Survey examines popularity of real-ear probe-microphone measures. Hear J 2010;63(5):27–28,30,32

5 Pediatric Audiology

● Introduction

A pediatric audiologist's main role is to identify and treat childhood hearing loss as young as possible. To do so, conventional testing techniques must be adapted to accommodate to the developmental level of the child. This chapter will review ways to identify hearing loss at a very young age and will describe specialized techniques used with children.

As children are continually developing, the successful pediatric audiologist is required to monitor development as well as diagnose and treat hearing loss. This includes tracking speech and language development, supporting academic accommodations, monitoring emotional and social development, educating parents on these topics, and referring to other specialists when concerns arise related to learning difficulties, cognitive delays, and/ or motor delays. The pediatric audiologist works as a part of a multidisciplinary team to best serve children with hearing loss.

Pediatric audiologists have special training in child development, counseling, behavior management, and pediatric specific testing techniques. Most pediatric facilities work with patients from birth through 18 to 21 years of age. Many pediatric facilities will continue to serve patients into their adult years if a significant developmental delay prevents the individual from participating in adult testing techniques.

● What Is Universal Newborn Hearing Screening?

Newborn infant hearing screening (NIHS) was recommended by National Institutes of Health consensus in 1993.[1] The concept gained traction when supported by a position statement from the American Academy of Pediatrics in 1999.[2] In 2007, the Joint Committee on Infant Hearing recommended that infants be screened for hearing loss by 1 month of age. If an infant refers on the screening, he/she should be referred for a diagnostic evaluation that is to be completed by 3 months of age. If hearing loss is identified at the diagnostic evaluation, the infant should begin intervention by 6 months of age.[3] As of 2008, 43 states have legislation requiring NIHS.[4]

Although each state's requirements differ, the Center for Disease Control (CDC) reports that in 2013 more than 90% of babies born in the United States were screened for hearing loss by 1 month of age and by 3 months of age greater than 95% had been screened. Screening tools and protocols vary from center to center; although, commonly used screening tools include automated auditory brainstem response (AABR) and otoacoustic emissions (OAE) testing (**Figs. 5.1** and **5.2**). Depending on the testing protocol that is implemented, the sensitivity and specificity of the screening can vary. For example, if OAE testing is the only screening used, neural hearing losses will be missed (i.e., hearing loss secondary to deficient auditory nerve or auditory neuropathy spectrum disorder). Regardless of the chosen screening tool, it is accepted that the screenings will miss the detection of mild hearing loss, sloping hearing loss when normal to mild hearing thresholds are present between ~1,000 and 3,000 Hz, and progressive hearing losses that worsen with time. Expected referral rates differ depending on the nursery level (i.e., well baby nursery versus neonatal intensive care unit [NICU]). For example, a well-baby nursery should have a refer rate between 0.5 and 2%, whereas a NICU may be near 10%. When combining across nursery levels, an overall refer rate of 4% is expected.[3]

The goal of NIHS is to identify hearing loss at a very young age to provide intervention prior to the child falling behind in language development. To

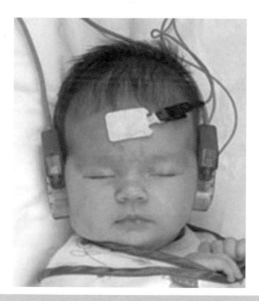

Fig. 5.1 An infant hearing screening performed with automated auditory brainstem response.[5]

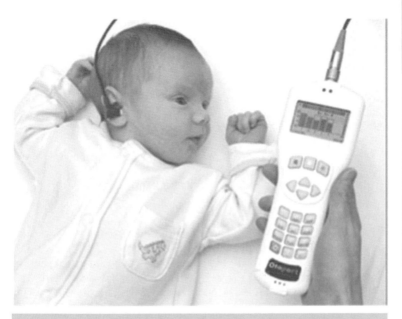

Fig. 5.2 An infant hearing screening performed with otoacoustic emissions.[6]

this end, most states have early intervention programs that monitor the screening data and support intervention resources (early hearing detection and identification). While national data suggest that newborn hearing screenings are successfully being implemented, the CDC reports that ~40% of the babies who are referred for diagnostic evaluation based on newborn hearing screening are lost to follow-up.[4] State programs are partnering with health professionals to improve this statistic.

● What Are the Risk Factors for Childhood Hearing Loss?

There are many risk factors associated with childhood hearing loss. Children with one or more risk factors should be referred for audiologic evaluation by 12 months of age and be closely monitored, even if they passed their NIHS. Parents should be made aware of these risk factors and counseled on the importance of follow-up care. Early identification is necessary to ensure that these infants receive medical intervention, hearing assistive devices, and access to therapeutic services as soon as possible. The following risk factors have been identified by the U.S. Department of Health and Human Services Centers for Disease Control and Prevention[7]:

- Caregiver concern regarding hearing, speech, language, or developmental delay.
- Family history of permanent childhood hearing loss.
- NICU stay of more than 5 days or any of the following regardless of length of stay:
  - Extracorporeal membrane oxygenation
  - Assisted ventilation
  - Exposure to ototoxic medications (gentamicin and tobramycin)
  - Loop diuretics (furosemide/Lasix)
  - Hyperbilirubinemia requiring exchange transfusion
- In utero infections, such as cytomegalovirus, herpes, rubella, syphilis, and toxoplasmosis.
- Craniofacial anomalies, including those involving the pinna, ear canal, ear tags, ear pits, and temporal bone anomalies.
- Physical findings, known to be associated with a permanent or conductive hearing loss. (e.g., a white forelock is associated with Waardenburg syndrome, which is associated with permanent hearing loss).
- Syndromes associated with hearing loss or progressive or late-onset hearing loss, such as neurofibromatosis, osteopetrosis, and Usher syndrome. Other frequently identified syndromes include Alport, Pendred, and Jervell and Lange-Nielson.
- Neurodegenerative disorders, such as Hunter syndrome, or sensory motor neuropathies, such as Friedreich ataxia and Charcot–Marie–Tooth syndrome.
- Culture-positive postnatal infections associated with sensorineural hearing loss, including confirmed bacterial and viral (especially herpes viruses and varicella) meningitis.
- Head trauma, especially basal skull/temporal bone fracture requiring hospitalization.
- Chemotherapy.
- Middle ear disorders such as:
  - Otitis media
  - Cholesteatoma
  - Tympanic membrane perforation
- Acoustic trauma.

● When Should Children Have Hearing Screening Beyond NIHS?

In addition to NIHS, children (even those without risk factors for hearing loss) should be screened for hearing loss throughout childhood to capture acquired hearing loss that was not present at birth. The American Speech–Language–Hearing Association (ASHA)[8] recommends a hearing screening schedule for school-age children as follows:

- Entry to preschool (~ 3 years of age)
- Annually from kindergarten through third grade (~ 5–9 years of age)
- Seventh grade (~ 12–13 years of age)
- Eleventh grade (~ 16–17 years old)

● What Test Methods Are Used to Evaluate Infant Hearing?

The ASHA recommends that the testing of infants (birth to 5 months of age) should rely primarily on physiologic measures of auditory function.[8] These measures include ABR (Chapter 2) using frequency-specific stimuli to estimate the audiogram, OAEs, and acoustic immittance measures (Chapter 2).[8,9] It should be noted that while conventional tympanometry (using a 226 Hz probe tone) is an effective tool in identifying middle ear dysfunction for children and adults (Chapter 2), high-frequency tympanometry (using a 1,000 Hz probe tone) has been proven to more accurately identify middle ear pathology in infants less than 7 months of age. This has been attributed to the acoustical and anatomical properties of the infants' external and middle ear system.[10] While OAEs and ABR can provide an objective estimate of hearing sensitivity, these diagnostic tests do not provide a direct measure of functional hearing abilities.[9] Therefore, behavioral hearing testing should always be attempted once the child is developmentally able to participate.

By 6 months developmental age, most infants can be conditioned to provide a behavioral response when an auditory stimulus is presented. Indicators that a child is ready for this type of testing include being able to sit up mostly unassisted and looking around the environment with curiosity. Visual reinforcement audiometry (VRA) is a diagnostic procedure used to evaluate hearing in infants between 6 and 30 months of age (**Fig. 5.3**). The infant is conditioned to turn his/her head toward a reinforcer (i.e., a toy/animal that lights up; a short video clip) each time the auditory stimulus is presented. Stach and Ramachandran[9] outline how this procedure is completed:

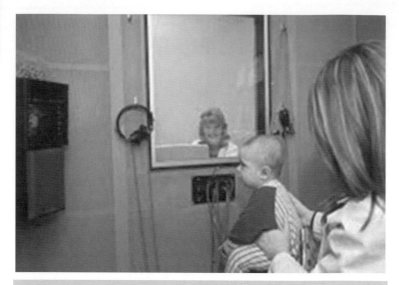

Fig. 5.3 Child participating in visual reinforcement audiometry testing.[11]

- Seat child in high chair, in a child's chair, or on a parent's lap.
- The test assistant or parent keeps the child's attention facing forward using quiet toys.
- The auditory stimulus is presented at a comfortably loud level above expected threshold. The auditory stimulus and conditioning/reinforcing toy remain on simultaneously for 3 to 4 seconds.
- Step three is repeated until the child consistently turns to the auditory stimulus.
- When the child is conditioned to respond, the auditory stimulus is presented without activating the conditioning/reinforcing toy. If the child turns toward the sound, the reinforcing toy is activated and conditioning is complete.
- Testing proceeds to obtain hearing thresholds for one low (500 Hz) and one high (2,000 Hz) frequency stimulus. The stimulus is decreased until the child stops responding and is then once again increased to bracket threshold.
- Additional frequencies to be tested will be determined by the response to the initial frequencies tested.
- Testing can proceed using insert earphones, bone vibrator, and hearing assistive technology (hearing aids, cochlear implants [CI], and frequency modulated [FM] systems).
- The reinforcing toy is activated only when the child makes a conditioned head turn to a sound. When in doubt, do not activate the reinforcer.

A test assistant or centering toy is critical in making sure the infant's attention is focused forward before the audiologist presents the stimulus so a head turn can be observed. It is also important that the infant's parent does not cue the infant when the auditory stimulus is presented. If this is observed, the test assistant or audiologist provides further instruction to the parent.

While testing in the sound-field is often necessary in the pediatric population due to limited acceptance of headphones or insert earphones, there are several considerations requiring attention. These include controlling and calibrating the test environment (minimizing ambient noise levels and positioning the patient at a calibrated location that takes into account distance and angle in relation to the loudspeaker, avoidance of standing waves) and interpreting results with caution due to the lack ear specific information. Sound-field testing must take place in a sound treated booth to minimize the ambient noise. Additionally, the space must be large enough to minimize the effects of reverberation and standing waves, which can invalidate results.

"In a reverberant space, the sound perceived by a listener is a combination of direct and reverberant sound. The ratio of direct sound is dependent on the distance between the source and the listener, and upon the reverberation time in the room. At a certain distance the two will be equal. This is called the 'critical distance.'" To further reduce the risk of standing waves, it is necessary to use warble tones or narrow band noise rather than pure tones during sound-field testing.[12] In addition to distance, the child's angle in relation to the loudspeaker must also be calibrated and observed during testing. Most commonly the child is either facing the speaker (0 degrees azimuth), or the speaker is off to the right or left of the child by 45 or 90 degrees azimuth (**Fig. 5.4**). Therefore, it is crucial that the patient is positioned correctly in the sound booth at the "critical distance" and calibrated angle to the loudspeaker to provide the accurate threshold level the patient is responding to.

It is also important to recognize that auditory thresholds obtained in the sound-field are not a reflection of the softest sounds a child can hear, but are actually the softest sounds a child can detect against the background noise in the test environment.[14] As a result, the American National Standards Institute (ANSI) has created standards specifically addressing maximum permissible ambient noise levels for testing to audiometric zero. For details, refer to the ANSI standard for maximum permissible noise levels (ANSI 3S1–1999) and the ANSI standard for audiometric zero is ANSI S3.6–1996 (ANSI).[15]

While sound-field audiometry can provide valuable information regarding hearing sensitivity, it is impossible to discern ear specific information

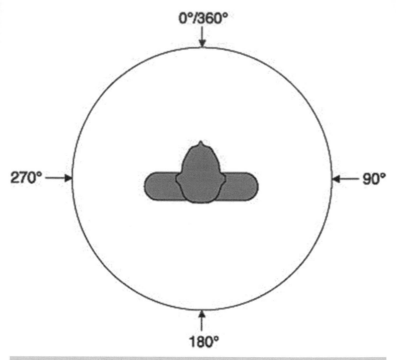

Fig. 5.4 Depiction of patient position when testing in the sound-field. Most commonly speakers are located at 0, 45, 90, 270, and 315 degrees.[13]

without the use of headphones or insert earphones. When thresholds are obtained in the sound-field, it should be known that those thresholds represent the better hearing ear. When headphones are not tolerated, parents are encouraged to practice wearing headphones with their child at home to help increase acceptance for future testing.

● What Test Methods Are Used for Toddlers and School-Aged Children?

Conditioned play audiometry is a diagnostic technique used for children with a developmental age of $2^1/_2$ to 5 years (**Fig. 5.5**). By $2^1/_2$ years of age, children can be conditioned to perform a motor task in response to a stimulus (i.e., drop a block in a bucket or put a ring on a stand when he/she hears a sound).[16] Some children will be able to participate in this method

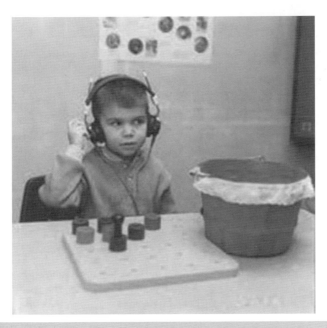

Fig. 5.5 Child participating in conditioned play audiometry testing.[17]

of testing slightly younger; however, reliability of responses may decline or attention may fatigue prior to the completion of an audiogram. At over 5 years of age, the child can participate in conventional audiometry, which consists of the child raising his/her hand or pushing a button in response to a tonal stimulus (Chapter 2).

For younger children, testing often begins in the sound-field (i.e., using loudspeakers) since headphones may not initially be accepted. The stimulus is presented at a level that is easily heard by the child to reinforce the response. "Hand-over-hand" is a technique that is used to condition children. The test assistant will put a toy in the child's hand and place his/her hand over the child's hand. When the stimulus is presented, the assistant will say, "We heard it, we put it in," and move the child's hand to perform the task (i.e., dropping a block into a bucket). The assistant will continue hand-over-hand until the child starts to respond independently when the stimulus is presented.[16]

Many times a speech awareness threshold (SAT) will be the first measure obtained since children condition most easily to a speech command (i.e., "put it in"). An SAT is the lowest intensity level in dB HL that the child can detect a speech stimulus for at least 50% of given presentations (it does not indicate recognition of the words/sounds spoken). For older children, repeating spondee words (i.e., two syllable words with equal stress on each syllable; includes such words as baseball, cowboy, hotdog, etc.), or pointing to the picture of a word that was presented can also provide a speech recognition/reception threshold (SRT) (**Fig. 5.6**). An SRT is the lowest intensity level in dB HL that the child can repeat the spondee word correctly for at least 50% of given presentations. Test order will vary depending on the suspected type of hearing loss. For example, for a child suspected of having a conductive hearing loss (i.e., abnormal tympanometry results), responses to a high-frequency tone (such as 2,000 Hz) should be obtained, as low frequencies are more impacted by the presence of otitis media. Once a high-frequency threshold is obtained, a low frequency is then evaluated (500 Hz). If sensorineural hearing loss is being ruled out (i.e., normal tympanometry), a low-frequency tone may be attempted first, since hearing tends to be better in the lower frequencies.[16] The audiologist then needs to determine what test information is most valuable to obtain. If a loss is identified via air-conduction testing at a low and high pitch and cooperation is a concern, the audiologist may choose to pursue bone-conduction testing prior to obtaining more pitches via air conduction to ascertain the type of hearing loss. If continued participation is not a concern, the audiologist will need to assess how likely the patient will tolerate headphones or insert earphones to pursue ear-specific information.

Frequencies 500 to 4,000 Hz are the primary focus, as those frequencies carry the majority of important speech information (250 Hz and 8,000 Hz are also tested if the child is still providing reliable responses). For younger

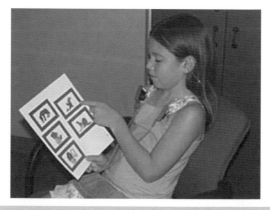

Fig. 5.6 Child completing an speech recognition/reception threshold task by pointing to pictures.[18]

children, the audiologist may choose not to present the stimulus below 10 and 15 dB HL (i.e., level of normal hearing). It is important to obtain as much diagnostic information as possible before the child fatigues. If the audiologist is consistently obtaining responses at 10 to 15 dB HL, the child's hearing is considered normal at that frequency and another frequency can be evaluated. For older compliant children, headphones may be placed at the start of testing and hearing thresholds can be obtained at each ear. While the goal is to obtain ear-specific information, if the child has an adverse reaction to headphones, testing can be completed in sound-field. Determining hearing sensitivity for at least the better ear provides important information, especially for a patient population first acquiring speech and language skills. If hearing is normal for at least one ear, that is adequate for speech and language development to begin.[19]

In addition to pure-tone audiometry, speech audiometry should also be evaluated beyond an SAT or SRT. Speech perception measures include the presentation of 25 to 50 developmentally appropriate words at an intensity level that is loud but comfortable (typically ~ 40 dB above the child's SAT or SRT). These words are presented sequentially to the child who either chooses the correct word from a set of four to six pictures (closed set) or repeats the word (open set) if speech production is intelligible. Speech perception measures allow the audiologist to quantify the clarity of speech sounds via percent of correctly identified words or phonemes (individual speech sounds) and provides additional information beyond audibility of sound. Speech perception measures should be obtained on all children and are critical for any child identified with a sensorineural hearing loss to help determine appropriate options for amplification.[9] If, however, tympanometry and the air conduction audiogram are abnormal (a temporary conductive hearing loss is suspected), the audiologist may choose to defer speech perception testing until the ears are clear and hearing has improved. See **Table 5.1** for a description of speech perception tests that are commonly used for the pediatric population and at which ages these tests should be performed when a child has normal speech and language development.

● How Do Audiometric Masking Methods Differ in Children Compared with Adults?

The goal of a diagnostic hearing test is to determine the type, magnitude, and configuration of hearing loss for each ear. To accurately assess

Table 5.1 A listing of speech perception tests and descriptions commonly used with the pediatric population[9]

Test	Language age	Description
Early Speech Perception Test[20]	Two years (or when the child is able to choose between two alternatives)	Closed-set pattern perception, spondee identification and monosyllable identification. This test is offered in a low verbal and standard version based on age and receptive vocabulary level of the child.
Northwestern University-Children's Perception of Speech[21]	> 2 and < 5 years	Closed-set picture pointing word recognition test with a vocabulary level appropriate for children ages 3 to 6 years.
Word Intelligibility by Picture Identification[22]	> 4 and < 8 years	Closed-set picture pointing speech recognition test and is commonly used for patients 5 years of age or older who may have articulation errors.
Phonetically Balanced Kindergarten–50 words[23]	> 5 and < 8 years	Open-set phonetically balanced monosyllabic word list. Presented live-voice or recorded.

auditory function for each ear, proper masking techniques may be required. Masking allows the audiologist to isolate responses from the test ear (TE) by introducing noise to the non-test ear (NTE). This eliminates the possibility of the signal crossing over and eliciting a response from the NTE (Chapter 2).

The most common masking procedure is called the "plateau method." "The masking plateau begins at the intensity at which the threshold in the TE remains stable when the masking noise in the NTE is increased."[24] It should be noted that there is not one universally accepted protocol for masking. Turner[24] proposed that testing begin with an initial masking level of 10 dB above the air-conduction threshold of the NTE (i.e., 10 dB sensation level [SL]). The threshold of the TE is reestablished and masking noise (via narrow band noise stimulus) is increased another 10 dB. Once the masking plateau has been achieved, that is, when two consecutive 10 dB increases in masking is introduced without an observed shift in threshold of the TE, the response is documented on the audiogram.[24]

Other protocols call for an initial level of masking of 15 dB above the air-conduction threshold of the NTE (i.e., 15 dB SL) and three consecutive 5 dB increases for plateau to be reached.[25] The same masking procedure is utilized for bone-conduction testing; however, correction factors of 20 dB at 250 Hz, 15 dB at 500 Hz, and 5 dB at 1,000 Hz need to be added to account for the occlusion effect if supra-aural headphones are used. A correction factor of 10 dB at 250 Hz is needed if insert earphones are being used.[26]

While the plateau method has been widely accepted as best practice for adult patients, pediatric audiologists often use a different approach. Masking can be very challenging and confusing for children. Some children have limited acceptance of the bone vibrator and retesting threshold multiple times while slowly increasing masking noise to the NTE to an effective level is not efficient. Instead of the plateau method, pediatric audiologists will often calculate the level of effective masking needed at the test frequency and present that level to the NTE. Once a response has been reliably obtained and repeated, the threshold of the TE and the masking level of the NTE will be recorded on the audiogram. By putting the effective masking level into the NTE when beginning testing, fewer responses are needed and more information can be obtained in one session. It is critical to determine effectively and efficiently the type of hearing loss so that medical management and treatment can be expedited.

● What Can Be Done If the Child Does Not Cooperate with Testing?

There are many techniques to entice a child to be cooperative with testing. There are times, however, that despite every attempt to encourage participation, testing cannot be completed. In those cases, if the child is compliant and has normal tympanograms, OAEs can be measured to provide some information on how the cochlea is functioning and a follow-up hearing test can be scheduled for another day. If information regarding hearing sensitivity is needed and cannot be reliably obtained, a sedated ABR should be considered.

Listed below are common procedures that may encourage participation.[16]

- Offer choices.
  - Offering choices is an excellent method to allow the child to feel he/she has control over the situation and encourage participation. For example, "Would you like to the play the piggy bank game or the ring game?"
- Change the game.
  - If the child's participation starts to decline, changing games may help maintain his/her interest and allow the audiologist to obtain additional diagnostic information.
- Positive reinforcement.
  - Positive reinforcement and praise should also be used generously throughout the test session. Examples include, "I really like the way you're listening, great job!" "That's the way to do it! Good work!"
- Take a break.
  - Allow the child to take a break, walk around or get a drink of water before trying again. Changing test booths and assistants may also be helpful.
- Ask the parent or siblings to step-out.
  - Sometimes children perform better when their parents are absent. Asking a parent to leave the room may allow you to refocus the child on the task the audiologist is asking the child to do.
  - If siblings are present and seem to be distracting, the audiologist may also ask the sibling step-out of the test booth as well.
- Reward.
  - Rewarding a child's behavior is an effective way to increase cooperation. Rewards may include stickers, food (fruit snacks, cheerios) candy, etc. VRA reinforcers may also be used to support a play task.
- Practice at home.
  - If a child refuses to wear headphones, parents are counseled to practice wearing headphones at home to increase tolerance when he/she returns for further testing.

● When Should a Child Be Referred for a Diagnostic Hearing Evaluation?

A child should complete a hearing evaluation for the following reasons:

- Referral on NIHS (up to three re-screens are allowed).[3]
- Referral on hearing screening.
- Caregivers or teachers are concerned about hearing abilities.
- Speech and/or language development is delayed.
- Child has one or more risk factors discussed earlier for childhood hearing loss.

It should be noted that no child is ever too young for a comprehensive hearing evaluation. See **Table 5.2** for a list of testing methods most commonly used at various developmental ages.

Table 5.2 Test methods for audiologic evaluation at various ages

Age of the child	Primary test method	Supporting test methods
Birth to 3 months	Sleep-deprived ABR	Otoscopy 1,000 Hz tympano-metry OAEs Middle ear reflexes
3–6 months (or older children who are unable to complete behavioral testing due to developmental or behavioral delay)	Sedated ABR	Otoscopy 1,000 Hz tympanome-try (under 6 months of age) 250 Hz tympanometry (over 6 months of age) OAEs Middle ear reflexes
6–24 months	Behavioral testing: VRA	Otoscopy 250 Hz tympanometry OAEs Middle ear reflexes
2–5 years	Behavioral testing: CPA	Otoscopy 250 Hz tympanometry Speech perception testing Middle ear reflexes
≥ 6 years	Behavioral testing: con-ventional audiometry	Otoscopy 250 Hz tympanometry Speech perception testing Middle ear reflexes

Abbreviations: ABR, auditory brainstem response; VRA, visual reinforcement audiome-try; CPA, conditioned play audiometry; OAEs, otoacoustic emissions.

● How Does Hearing Loss Impact Children?

When hearing loss presents itself during childhood, it can impact several domains. Per ASHA,[27] areas most notably impacted include the following:

- Auditory, speech and language development
- Academic achievement
- Socialization
- Self-concept/identity

For children with pre- or perilingual onset of hearing loss, the most obvious effect from hearing loss is the delay in speech and language acquisition. Often this is not noticed until the child is between 15 and 18 months of age and is not talking; although, there are precursors that can identify hearing loss sooner. It is important to know typical developmental milestones to identify a delay. **Table 5.3** provides a list of auditory, speech, and language developmental milestones.[28]

Often when hearing loss is diagnosed at a young age and effectively treated, hearing-impaired children can develop speech and language at the same pace as their normal-hearing peers. There are, however, some speech and

Table 5.3 Auditory, speech, and language milestones for typically developing children with normal hearing[28]

Birth to 3 months	• Startles to loud sounds. • Stills or smiles when spoken to. • Calms to caregivers voice if upset. • When feeding, starts or stops sucking in response to sound. • "Coos" and makes pleasure sounds. • Has different cries signifying different needs. • Smiles when he/she sees you.
4–6 months	• Follows sound with his/her eyes. • Responds to changes in tone of caregiver's voice. • Notices toys that make sound. • Pays attention to music. • Babbles in speech-like way and uses many different sounds that begin with /p/, /b/, /m/. • Laughs. • Babbles when excited or happy. • Makes gurgling sounds when alone or playing with caregiver.
7 months–1 year	• Enjoys playing peek-a-boo and pat-a-cake. • Turns and looks in the direction of sounds. • Listens when spoken to. • Understands words for common items such as "cup," "shoe," or "juice." • Responds to requests such as "come here." • Babbles using long and short groups of vowels ("tata," "upup," "bibibi"). • Babbles to get and keep attention. • Communicates using gestures such as waving or holding arms up. • Imitates different speech sounds. • Has one or two words ("hi," "dog," "dada," or "mama") by first birthday.

1–2 years	• Knows a few parts of the body and can point to them when asked. • Follows simple commands ("roll the ball"). • Understands simple questions ("Where are your shoes?"). • Enjoys simple stories, rhymes, and songs. • Points to pictures when named in a book. • Acquires new words regularly. • Uses some one- or two-word questions ("where kitty?" or "Go bye bye?"). • Puts two words together ("more cookie"). • Uses many different consonant sounds at the beginning of words.
2–3 years	• Has a word for almost everything. • Uses two- to three-word phrases to talk about and ask for things. • Uses /k/, /g/, /f/, /t/, /d/, and /n/ sounds. • Speaks in a way that is understood by family and friends. • Names objects to ask for them or to direct attention to them.
3–4 years	• Hears you when you call from another room. • Prefers the sound level of the TV or radio at a similar level to the rest of a normal-hearing family. • Answers simple "who?" "what?" "where?" "why?" questions. • Talks about activities at day care, preschool, and friends' homes. • Uses sentences with four or more words. • Speaks easily without repeating syllables or words.
4–5 years	• Pays attention to a short story and answers questions about it. • Hears and understands most of what is said at home and school. • Uses sentences that give many details. • Tells stories that stay on topic. • Communicates easily with other children and adults. • Says most sounds correctly except for a few (/l/, /s/, /r/, /v/, /z/, /ch/, /sh/, and /th/ may be hard). • Begins rhyming words. – Names some letters and numbers. • Uses adult grammar.

language difficulties that are common to children with hearing impairment and may persist despite treatment. These difficulties will require ongoing therapy. The ASHA[27] outlines areas of difficulty as follows:
• Vocabulary may develop more slowly.

- Concrete words (e.g., cat, jump, red) are gained more readily than abstract words (e.g., before, jealous, equal) and function words (e.g., the, an, are, a).
- There is difficulty understanding words with more than one meaning (e.g., "bank is a place where you store money and a edge of a stream").
- Produce shorter and simpler sentences with difficulty expanding.
- Omitting endings of words or inaccurately substituting other speech sounds at the end of words. This can affect speech production and lead to errors with grammatical markers (possessive/plural /s/), subject and verb agreement, and verb tense (/ed/ endings).
- Soft sounds can be difficult to hear (/s/sh/f/t/k/). This can lead to misunderstanding and poor speech production.

As the child moves into a classroom setting, academic achievement can also be negatively affected without good sound access and communication skills. This can be as subtle as appearing inattentive when background noise is present and as significant as not being able to learn new vocabulary or access curriculum. In addition to academic concerns, the hearing-impaired child may become socially isolated if he/she is unable to successfully communicate with peers. If not addressed, this can lead to depression and low self-esteem. It is not uncommon for hearing-impaired children to gravitate toward adults to act as "peers." Adults may be more tolerant of speech/language mistakes and more patient and attentive to the child's needs when communicating. As self-concept and identity develop, particularly in adolescents, it is common for hearing-impaired children to wonder why they are different, especially if they are only surrounded by hearing peers. It can be helpful to introduce these children to peers with hearing loss throughout childhood. At times, counseling services may be beneficial.[27]

● What Is Auditory Neuropathy Spectrum Disorder and How Does It Present Itself in a Child?

Auditory neuropathy spectrum disorder (ANSD), commonly known as auditory dysynchrony, is a term used to describe a disorder of the auditory system characterized by an absent ABR, present OAE and/or cochlear microphonic, absent acoustic reflex thresholds, poor speech perception, and varying degrees of hearing loss as indicated via behavioral hearing testing. In general, it is understood that the auditory pathway through the level of the outer hair cells (OHCs) is functioning properly, with the breakdown occurring somewhere beyond the inner hair cells (IHCs) as the signal travels along the auditory nerve and through the brainstem. In cases of ANSD, there are no audiologic tools to differentiate site of lesion beyond the OHCs. It is impossible, therefore, based on physiologic tests, to fully isolate a sensory (IHC loss) from synaptic dysfunction from a neural hearing loss (axonal loss or dysynchrony due to demyelination). In addition, dysfunction can exist at more than one site along the auditory pathway.[29]

In terms of presentation, hearing sensitivity ranges in ANSD from normal to profound and often has a flat or reverse-slope audiometric configuration. Hearing sensitivity may fluctuate and can be progressive for some children. Speech perception is often substantially poorer than would be predicted from the audiogram. Further, speech perception in the presence of background noise can be significantly impaired.[29]

Treatment includes conventional amplification, FM systems, or CI. Since ANSD varies significantly in terms of hearing sensitivity, functional outcomes and treatment options vary considerably as well.

● What Is Central Auditory Processing Disorder and How Does It Present in a Child?

A central auditory processing disorder (CAPD) is the inability, or the impaired ability, to attend to, discriminate, recognize, or comprehend information presented auditorily in children with normal hearing sensitivity and normal intelligence. "It is important to emphasize that CAPD is an auditory deficit that is not the result of a higher-order, more global deficit such as autism, intellectual disabilities, attention deficits, or similar impairments."[30]

Common characteristics exhibited by a child having a central auditory processing disorder include the following:
• Difficulty listening in background noise
• Difficulty following directions
• Exhaustion from listening in class
• Reading and/or spelling difficulties
• Difficulty with phonics and speech sound recognition
• Poor auditory memory
• Often misunderstands what is said and needs information to be repeated

- Poor expressive language skills
- Slow or delayed response to verbal requests and instructions
- Poor auditory attention
- Difficulty learning through the auditory channel[30]

In order for a CAPD evaluation to be completed, the child must have normal peripheral hearing sensitivity, normal cognitive function (Full Scale IQ of 85 or above), and must be at least 7 years of age. For children younger than 7 years, there is excessive variability in brain function impeding an accurate diagnosis of CAPD. A multidisciplinary team approach is also important to provide a comprehensive view of the child's present level of functioning. Team members may include the child's parent, teacher, neuropsychologist/ psychologist, speech-language pathologist, and audiologist. The child's parent can provide important case history information including birth history, previous and current health concerns, speech and language development, auditory and communicative difficulties, educational history including services and accommodations, social development, previous therapies, etc. A teacher can provide valuable insight in behavioral and learning observations, as well as information on how the child is performing academically. A neuropsychologist/ psychologist may evaluate cognitive functioning, memory, and academic performance to determine whether a learning disability is present and identify other factors (e.g., attention, visual processing, etc.) that may be contributing to the child's difficulties. A speech-language pathologist can provide an assessment of expressive and receptive language abilities, which is essential to appropriately interpret CAPD results. The speech-language pathologist is also the professional that most often provides therapy to strengthen auditory processing skills when deficits are identified. The audiologist is responsible for evaluating the child's peripheral auditory system, determining/executing an appropriate test battery to assess the child's central auditory system, and assists in developing an intervention plan. While input from all team members is extremely important; the diagnosis of CAPD can only be made by an audiologist through a series of tests targeting different auditory processing areas.

To evaluate a child for CAPD, a comprehensive assessment of the child's peripheral and central auditory system must be completed. An assessment of the peripheral auditory system should include pure-tone audiometry, speech perception measures, OAEs, and immittance testing prior to the administration of the CAPD test battery. It is important to verify that hearing sensitivity and middle ear function are normal as hearing loss or fluid in the middle ear can impact performance on tests that aim to isolate central auditory function.

At present, there is not a universally accepted CAPD test protocol. While electrophysiological tests, such as middle latency responses and the P300, have been used in assessment of auditory processing disorders, this section will focus on behavioral tests of central auditory processing. The two most commonly used models for diagnosis and classification of CAPD include the Bellis/Ferre model[31] and the Buffalo model.[32] Regardless of the model, it is well accepted that the battery includes behavioral tests of central auditory processing in the following categories:[30,31,32]

- *Dichotic listening tests:* Dichotic listening refers to the condition in which both ears receive differing signals simultaneously or in an overlapping manner via independent channels delivered under earphones. Test stimuli may include numbers, sentences, words, or nonsense syllables. The more similar the acoustic qualities of the stimuli and the more overlap that is present in timing between ears, the more difficult the task will be. The child is asked to either repeat everything that is heard across both ears (referred to as divided attention or binaural integration), or repeat only what is heard in one particular ear (referred to as directed attention or binaural separation). A child with CAPD is likely to have difficulty with binaural integration and binaural separation tasks as compared with test norms provided for typically developing age-matched peers.[33]

- *Monaural low-redundancy tests:* These measures require the child to listen to a degraded speech signal in one ear and repeat back what is heard, with both the right and left ears being tested separately. Spoken language has many redundant patterns, which allow listeners to fill in missing pieces of a signal when necessary. These predictive features of speech are referred to as extrinsic redundancy and lead to predictability. Extrinsic redundancy arises from multiple and overlapping acoustic and linguistic cues that are carried by common phoneme combinations, prosody of speech, syntactic and semantic cues. For example, certain phoneme combinations are often paired together to form words while other combinations are unacceptable or uncommon. Additionally, the sentence structure is governed by grammatical rules, and word order or word choice is supported by sentence context. A sentence stimulus, therefore, would be considered the most redundant signal and a nonsense syllable would be considered the least redundant or very unpredictable. Additionally, the central auditory nervous system (CANS) has intrinsic redundancy built in for further support. The CANS has multiple parallel pathways (ipsilateral and contralateral to the listening ear) carrying information bottom-up and top-down. If the extrinsic redundancy of the incoming signal is reduced and the intrinsic redundancy of the CANS is not properly functioning, a child will have difficulty understanding the degraded signal. For this test measure, the incoming sentence or word stimulus is degraded in some way (e.g., by changing the frequency or spectral content, adding time-compression, applying low-pass filters, or adding background noise or reverberation). The child is then asked to repeat the degraded signal by filling in the blanks or repairing the stimulus. A child with CAPD may have difficulty with this task, scoring significantly below the provided test norms for age-matched typically developing peers.[33]

- *Temporal processing tests:* Temporal processing is necessary to discern subtle auditory cues. In speech perception, temporal processing allows a listener to discriminate similar words (e.g., dime vs. time or boots vs. boost). Temporal processing is also necessary for the perception of music (i.e., order of notes, ascending or descending scale). Temporal processing can be tested in various ways including the following:
  - Detecting a gap or pause embedded within a sound stimuli. This can be performed in quiet and/or in background noise.
  - Sequencing pitch patterns of tonal stimuli (e.g., hearing three tones sequentially that are one of two pitches (high pitch or low pitch) and labeling the pattern as applies. For example, high-low-high; low-low-high, etc.).
  - Reporting duration patterns of tonal stimuli (e.g., hearing three tones sequentially that are one of two lengths (long duration or short duration) of presentation and labeling the pattern as applies. For example, long-short-long.).

Children with CAPD may score significantly lower than their age-matched typically developing peers per test norms on these measures. It is also possible that they may be able to discern the auditory differences (particularly on the pitch or duration sequencing activities) but are only be able to report these perceptions by humming or with other motor gestures.[33]

- *Binaural interaction testing:* With this testing, two separate partial signals are presented sequentially to each ear; when combined the two stimuli create a whole message. The child must listen to the sequential stimuli and then repeat the message in its entirety by combining what was heard at each ear. Binaural interaction (or binaural fusion) differs from dichotic listening as the two stimuli are sequentially presented rather than simultaneously presented at each ear. A child with CAPD may have difficulty with this task, scoring significantly below the provided test norms for age-matched typically developing peers.[33]

Treatment for CAPD is highly individualized and generally focuses on three primary areas: environmental modifications (e.g., classroom placement, teaching and communication styles, use of an assistive listening device [Chapter 4], etc.), compensation strategies (e.g., visual presentation of the materials, relying on note-takers, pre-teaching new vocabulary and concepts, etc.), and direct remediation of the auditory deficit(s) via auditory training exercises. While further research is needed in the area of CAPD, it is evident that early diagnosis and treatment using a combination of top-down (e.g., metalinguistic and metacognitive skills), and bottom-up strategies (e.g., auditory training) is critical to maximize the neuroplasticity of the auditory system and strengthen auditory processing weaknesses.[33]

● Who Is on the Multidisciplinary Team That Treats Pediatric Hearing Loss?

To optimally serve a child with hearing impairment, a team of professionals must work together. Most commonly, team members include the following professionals who specialize in pediatric hearing loss:
- Otolaryngologist and nurse
- Audiologist
- Speech-language pathologist
- Developmental therapist for hearing-impaired (DT-H) (birth to 3 years of age)
- Deaf educator (≥ 3 years)
- Social worker
- Geneticist and genetic counselor
- Psychologist/neuropsychologist

Many children with hearing loss have additional developmental delay(s), a concurrent diagnosis, or a syndrome. It is, therefore, not uncommon to partner with additional professionals. These professionals include occupational therapy (OT), physical therapy (PT), neurology, opthamology, etc. To partner effectively with the team, all members must communicate regularly and work to coordinate services and counseling.

● What Are Various Communication Modalities That a Child with Hearing Impairment May Use and How Does a Family Choose the Optimal Path?

There are several ways to communicate with children. This is not a concept that is often considered for most typically developing children. Children hear language, process it, and begin to replicate it. It simply takes exposure to spoken language to make it happen. That concept can be true for hearing-impaired children as well. If hearing-impaired children have no other developmental concerns beyond hearing loss and can access language, they will begin to understand and replicate it. Because of the hearing loss, the team must think about the best way to provide access to language.

Table 5.4 provides a description of various communication modalities commonly used with hearing-impaired children.[34]

While the team provides information and education related to the child's abilities and possible communication modalities, the child's family is at the center of this decision as they must make a choice that promotes the family culture while simultaneously lending to success for the child. The professional's role is to educate the parent about the options, outline how to achieve success via each path, and support the family as they sort through the information. This can be a very overwhelming process for parents. A few concepts that can help a family in their decision include the following:

- A child will only learn at the proper rate if he/she is immersed in the chosen language. The family must be proficient and comfortable in the communication mode that is selected. Whatever choice is made becomes a commitment requiring energy and time (i.e., hearing aids/CI and spoken language or family/community learning sign language).
- The family and caregivers need to communicate consistently and constantly with the child.
- The child's hearing history, vision, learning/cognitive abilities, and current ability to perceive sound through amplification often guide the decision. Examples include the following:
  - If a child has profound hearing loss and is not a candidate for a CI, he/she will need some form of visual communication versus listening and speaking alone.
  - If a child is visually impaired, he/she may optimize communication by relying on hearing devices and speaking.

● How Are Pediatric Hearing Aid Fittings Different Than Adult Hearing Aid Fittings?

Children require optimal access to speech sounds in order learn new vocabulary and grammatical structures. Young children have not yet acquired comprehensive speech and language skills and have not yet mastered certain academic concepts; therefore, they cannot fill in the blanks as well as adults when something is not heard or is heard incorrectly. In fact, it is well documented that children need more sound access than adults, especially in the high-frequency region.[35,36]

Table 5.4 Communication modalities commonly used by patients with hearing impairment[34]

Communication modality	Description	Are hearing devices required?
Auditory–verbal	A child is taught to strictly rely on hearing to learn speech and language.	Yes
Auditory–oral	A child is taught to listen and speak but utilizes lip-reading and speech reading (gestures and facial expressions) as needed.	Yes
Cued speech	A child is taught to listen and speak, but the communication partner utilizes hand shapes near his or her mouth to help make sounds that are difficult to lip-read become more visual.	Yes
Simultaneous communication/TC	The child utilizes listening, speaking, and sign language to communicate. The sign language used is in English word order and often conceptual to support spoken communication.	Yes
Manual communication/ASL	The child utilizes sign language alone to communicate. ASL is a full language and has a sign for every language concept. It is a different language than English and has different word order and grammar. One cannot speak English and use ASL simultaneously.	Optional

Abbreviations: TC, total communication; ASL, American sign language.

Therefore, it is likely that pediatric fitting methods will include the use of DSL i/o prescriptive targets which provide increased gain, particularly in the high-frequency region when compared with an adult fitting (see Chapter 4 for more details on prescriptive targets).

In addition, while adaptive multichannel directional microphone technology is the default setting for adult patients in hearing aids (see Chapter 4 for detailed description of this technology), audiologists treating hearing loss in pediatric patients are more conflicted on whether to apply this algorithm.[37] While most agree this technology is advantageous because it improves speech perception and comfort in background noise, some are concerned that directional microphones will cause children to miss crucial communication/learning opportunities that occur beside or behind them.[37] Omnidirectional microphones allow the child to hear from all around rather than eliminating what is judged to be background noise or competing signals. Without the use of directional microphone algorithms one may be worried that background noise will be overwhelming. To combat background noise, it is common that children utilize a remote microphone system (FM system) to improve the SNR.[37]

With an FM system the primary speaker or group of speakers has access to a microphone that sends their voice(s) to a receiver. The receiver can deliver the signal in several ways: outputted via a speaker placed on the child's desk (personal sound-field system), outputted via a set of speakers strategically placed around the classroom (sound-field system), or outputted directly through the child's hearing aid(s) or CI(s) (personal system). This technology allows improved access to the primary speaker by maintaining the volume of a speech signal despite distance, by eliminating distortion caused by reverberation, and by adjusting the volume of the primary speaker to overcome the background noise detected in the environment.[37]

Other considerations for pediatric hearing aid fittings include the need for tamper resistant battery doors, disabling program buttons, enabling indicator lights, and providing listening stethosets (**Fig. 5.7**) for at home troubleshooting. These options will help keep the child safe, ensure that device settings are not accidently changed, and allow the parent to monitor device function. It is also the case that patients under the age of 18 years must have medical clearance from a physician with an audiogram measured within 6 months of the hearing aid fitting.

In addition, children grow at a rapid rate. It is therefore common to use a behind-the-ear (BTE) hearing aid (Chapter 4). This allows the audiologist to avoid recasing a custom hearing aid (i.e., in-the-ear, etc.) repeatedly to accommodate the child's growth. If this were done, the child would be without his/her hearing aids often while the devices are sent away for remake/repair. With a BTE hearing aid, the earmold is the only part that will need to be remade. The earmold can be detached from the hearing aid and exchanged as the child grows, thus giving children consistent sound access.

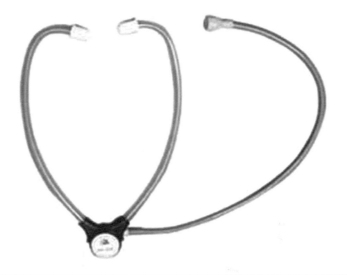

Fig. 5.7 A listening stethoset is shown in this picture. Caregivers can listen to a child's hearing aid with this tool to ensure proper function.[38]

● How Do Audiologists Verify Optimal Hearing Aid and CI Fittings and Track Progress for Children with Hearing Devices?

When optimizing a hearing device fitting and tracking progress over time for a child with hearing loss who utilizes assistive listening device(s), traditional hearing aid(s), bone anchored hearing aid(s), or CI(s) (Chapter 4), one must ensure the following:

- Audibility of speech sounds at an average and soft intensity level.
- Comfort to loud sounds in the environment.
- Maximum clarity of spoken words and sentences in quiet and in the presence of background noise.
- Appropriate speech and language progress as assessed by a speech-language pathologist every 6 to 12 months.

Additional information can be provided by the child, parent, and teacher via questionnaires. These questionnaires can provide valuable information regarding judgments pertaining to real-life performance and quality of life and may guide the audiologists fitting and programming decisions.

Examples of information commonly obtained through caregiver interview/ questionnaire include descriptions of the child's responses to sounds in the everyday environment, comfort/discomfort to loud sounds, changes in expressive and receptive language abilities and speech production, socialization patterns, a description of the child's willingness to wear devices, and quantification of device use. Subjective information may also serve as a counseling tool in helping to establish realistic and appropriate expectations.

● What Are Common Educational Accommodations and Services That a Child with Hearing Loss May Have?

Children with hearing loss qualify for educational services and support through federal laws that are implemented at the state level. For children less than 3 years of age, an individualized family service plan (IFSP) is provided.[39] The IFSP often provides resources for audiologic support (such as evaluation and hearing aids) and in home therapy/parent education from several professionals as deemed appropriate by the service coordinator. In addition to an audiologist, a DT-H and/or SLP is most commonly needed to support hearing-impaired children. It is not uncommon for an OT and PT to be provided as well if other developmental milestones are not being met.

For children 3 years and older, federal law requires children with hearing loss in the public school system to be supported by an individualized education plan (IEP) or a 504 Plan. The child must show a significant delay to qualify for an IEP. If an IEP is implemented, extra services and accommodations will be provided as determined by the team. If the child does not have significant developmental or academic delay but requires educational accommodations to support their hearing needs, they will be provided with a 504 Plan. A 504 Plan does not provide extra services, only accommodations.[39] Common services for school-aged children with hearing loss include instruction with a deaf educator, instruction with an SLP, and audiologic support. Common accommodations may include access to an assistive listening device to improve understanding in a noisy classroom (FM system), preferential seating, interpreter services, real-time captioning, access to a note-taker, access to curriculum prior to class, etc.

● Conclusions

Providing quality care to children with hearing impairment requires identification of hearing loss at a very young age, application of adapted evaluation and fitting techniques, an understanding of child development, and a
multidisciplinary team approach.

● Acknowledgment

Thank you to Kelly Taylor, Au.D., CCC-A for her significant contributions in
writing this chapter. Kelly is a pediatric audiologist at St. Louis Children's
Hospital who specializes in behavioral hearing evaluation, hearing aid care,
and CAPD.

References

1. Utah State University and National Center for Hearing Assessment and
    Management Staff. Early hearing detection and intervention (EHDI)
    legislation: overview. NCHAM. http://www.infanthearing.org/legisla-
    tion/. Published 1999. Last updated 2016. Accessed June 15, 2016
2. American Academy of Pediatrics (AAP). Newborn hearing screening
    and intervention. Pediatrics 1999;103(2):527–530
3. American Academy of Pediatrics, Joint Committee on Infant
    Hearing. Year 2007 position statement: principles and guidelines
    for early hearing detection and intervention programs. Pediatrics
    2007;120(4):898–921
4. Center for Disease Control (CDC). Annual data early hearing detection
    and intervention (EHDI) program. http://www.cdc.gov/ncbddd/hear-
    ingloss/ehdi-data.html. Updated 2013. Accessed June 15, 2016
5. Author unknown. Infant screening: automated auditory brainstem
    response.   http://www.health.utah.gov/cshcn/programs/ehdi.html.
    Accessed August 28, 2016
6. Author unknown. Infant screening: otoacoustic emissions test. http://
    www.infanthearing.org/screening/equipment.html. Accessed August
    28, 2016
7. Center for Disease Control (CDC). Hearing loss in infants and young
    children. http://www.cdc.gov/ncbddd/hearingloss/freematerials/pcp-
    hearing-loss.pdf. Accessed July 26, 2016

8. American Speech–Language–Hearing Association (ASHA) Panel on Audiologic Assessment. Guidelines for audiologic screening. American Speech–Language–Hearing Association. http://www.asha.org/policy/GL1997-00199/#sec1.2.1. Published 1997. Accessed June 15, 2016

9. Stach B, Ramachandran V. Hearing disorders in children. In: Madell J, Flexer C, eds. Pediatric Audiology: Diagnosis, Technology, and Management. New York, NY: Thieme; 2014:2(35–56)

10. Sood AS, Bons CS, Narang GS. High frequency tympanometry in neonates with normal otoacoustic emissions: measurements and interpretations. Indian J Otolaryngol Head Neck Surg 2013;65(3):237–243

11. Author unknown. Visual reinforcement audiometry. http://www.statenislandhearing.com/pediatric-evaluations. Accessed August 27, 2016

12. White G, Louie G. The Audio Dictionary. 3rd ed. Seattle: University of Washington Press; 2005:89

13. Dobie RA, Van Hemel S, eds. National Research Council (US) Committee on Disability Determination for Individuals with Hearing Impairments. Overhead view of listener. Determining Eligibility for Social Security Benefits (print). Washington, DC: National Academies Press; 2004

14. Berger E. Options in defining background noise during audiometric testing. http://multimedia.3m.com/mws/media/893208O/options-in-defining-background-noise-during-audiometric-testing.pdf. Published December 20, 2007. Accessed August 28, 2016

15. National Research Council (US) Committee on Disability Determination for Individuals with Hearing Impairments. In: Dobie R, Van Hemel S, eds. Hearing Loss: Determining Eligibility for Social Security Benefits. Washington, DC: National Academies Press; 2004. Appendix B, American National Standards on Acoustics. http://www.ncbi.nlm.nih.gov/books/NBK207830/. Accessed October 24, 2016

16. Madell J. Using conditioned play audiometry to test hearing in children older than 21/2 years. In: Madell J, Flexer C, eds. Pediatric Audiology: Diagnosis, Technology, and Management. New York, NY: Thieme; 2014:76–80

17. Unknown author. Conditioned play audiometry. http://www.hearing-testsjust4kidz.com/About-Hearing-Tests.html. Accessed August 27, 2016

18. Unknown author. Speech reception threshold via picture pointing task. http://www.statenislandhearing.com/pediatric-evaluations. Accessed August 27, 2016

19. McKay S. Unilateral hearing loss in children. American Speech–Language–Hearing Association. www.asha.org/public/hearing/Unilateral-hearing-loss-in-children/. Accessed August 27, 2016

20. Geers A, Moog J. Evaluating speech perception skills: tools for measuring benefits of cochlear implants, tactile aids, and hearing aids. In:

Owens E, Kessler D, eds. Cochlear Implants in Children. Boston, MA: College Hill Press; 1989:227–256

21. Elliott L, Katz J. Development of a New Children's Test of Speech Discrimination (Technical Manual). St Louis, MO: Auditec; 1980

22. Ross M, Lerman J. A picture identification test for hearing-impaired children. J Speech Hear Res 1970;13(1):44–53

23. Haskins H. A phonetically balanced test of speech discrimination for children. Unpublished master's thesis. 1949. Evanston, IL: Northwestern University

24. Turner RG. Masking redux. II: a recommended masking protocol. J Am Acad Audiol 2004;15(1):29–46

25. American Academy of Audiology Task Force. Audiology clinical practice guidelines: audiologic management of adult hearing impairment. Audiol Today 2006;18:5

26. Roeser R, Clark J. Clinical masking. Roeser R, Valente M, Hosford-Dunn H, eds. Audiology Diagnosis. New York, NY: Thieme; 2000:243–279

27. American Speech–Language–Hearing Association (ASHA). Effects of hearing loss on development. American Speech–Language–Hearing Association. Published 2015. Accessed June 15, 2016

28. United States Department of Health and Human Services. National Institutes of Health (NIH). National Institute of Deafness and Communication Disorders (NIDCD). Fact sheet: voice, speech and language; speech and language milestones. National Institute of Deafness and Communication Disorders (NIDCD). http://www.nidcd.nih.gov. Published September 2010. Updated December 2014. Accessed June 15, 2016

29. Norrix LW, Velenovsky DS. Auditory neuropathy spectrum disorder: a review. J Speech Lang Hear Res 2014;57(4):1564–1576

30. Bellis T. Understanding auditory processing disorders in children. American Speech–Language–Hearing Association. http://www.asha.org/public/hearing/disorders/understand-apd-child.htm. Accessed June 29, 2016

31. Bellis T. Overview of central tests. In: Bellis T, ed. Assessment and Management of Central Auditory Processing Disorders in the Educational Setting: From Science to Practice. 2nd ed. Clifton Park, NY: Delmar Cengage Learning; 2003:203

32. Katz J. Auditory processing disorder: evaluation to therapy, the Buffalo Model. Audiology Online. http://www.audiologyonline.com/articles/apd-evaluation-to-therapy-buffalo-945. Published May 14, 2007. Accessed August 28, 2016

33. Cunningham R. APD in children: a time compressed overview. Audiology Online. http://www.audiologyonline.com/articles/apd-in-children-time-compressed-11953. Published July 2013. Accessed August 27, 2016

34. Anderson K. Parents Know Webpage. Minnesota Department of Education. http://parentsknow.state.mn.us. Published 2011. Accessed June 15, 2016

35. Stelmachowicz PG, Pittman AL, Hoover BM, Lewis DE, Moeller MP. The importance of high-frequency audibility in the speech and language development of children with hearing loss. Arch Otolaryngol Head Neck Surg 2004;130(5):556–562

36. Stelmachowicz PG, Lewis DE, Choi S, Hoover B. Effect of stimulus bandwidth on auditory skills in normal-hearing and hearing-impaired children. Ear Hear 2007;28(4):483–494

37. McCreery R. Building blocks: directional microphone use with children: no straight answer. Hear J 2013;66(11):8–9

38. Unknown author. Stethoset. http://www.aliexpress.com/store/group/Listening-tube-Accessories/830007_503463662.html. Accessed August 27, 2016

39. United States Department of Education. Building the legacy: IDEA 2004. http://idea.ed.gov/. Published 2004. Accessed June 15, 2016

6   Doctoral Education in Audiology

● How Has Education in Audiology Evolved?

Audiology's professional roots date back to days following World War II, when veterans experienced blast trauma, noise-induced hearing loss, and other challenges. This new profession shared common threads with professions of otolaryngology, psychology, rehabilitation, speech-language pathology, and others. Audiology has evolved to the status enjoyed today, where audiologists play an instrumental role in prevention, assessment, and management of hearing loss. Audiologists treat patients across the entire lifespan, from newborn through geriatric populations. This age span is widening, as the infant mortality rate diminishes and as the country experiences the "graying of America," with Baby Boomers beginning to experience deficits in hearing acuity.

The scope of practice is ever expanding, including comprehensive diagnostic evaluation, evaluation of auditory processing disorders, tinnitus assessment and treatment, misophonia and hyperacusis assessment and treatment, hearing aid and cochlear implant evaluation and fitting, vestibular function testing, aural (re)habilitation, electrophysiologic assessment, intraoperative monitoring, hearing assistive technology, and much more. Educational requirements for audiology practice have also developed greatly, in line with professional growth. The Academy of Dispensing Audiologists promoted the concept of a clinical doctorate as the entry-level degree for audiology in 1988. The American Academy of Audiology (AAA) released a position paper in 1991 that supported the Doctor of Audiology (Au.D.) degree, along with a recommended framework for academic and clinical study. In 1992, the American Speech-Language-Hearing Association (ASHA) supported the Au.D. degree as the entry level degree for practice. Affiliated accreditation bodies engaged in much discussion and modified standards to which academic programs must adhere. Professional organizations mandated that the entry level for practice in 2007 was the Au.D. degree. ASHA mandated that audiologists seeking the Certificate of Clinical Competence (CCC) after January 1, 2007 must hold the Au.D. In similar fashion, the American Board of Audiology's (ABA) Certification, affiliated with the AAA, required a clinical doctoral degree as a prerequisite for application. Prior to that time, a master's degree was required, with graduates completing a clinical fellowship year under supervision, following graduation and prior to licensure and permanent employment.

• What Is Currently Involved in Au.D. Education?

The Au.D. is considered to be a clinically oriented doctoral degree and there are ~75 Au.D. programs in the United States. Some foreign countries have progressed to an Au.D. degree requirement to practice while most employ a bachelor's or master's degree model. There is a great variability among programs here in the United States and efforts have been initiated toward greater standardization, as well as overall assessment of the current model. While undergraduate students may apply to an Au.D. program from myriad backgrounds, most have an undergraduate foundation in the Speech and Hearing Sciences (SHS). Many undergraduate programs offer such majors or minors in SHS or Communication Sciences and Disorders, with graduates then seeking additional graduate education in speech-language pathology, audiology, or a similar field. While optimum undergraduate education for entering the audiology profession is still being considered, many agree that a heavy foundation in math and the sciences is beneficial. Some students who originally seek a premedicine major learn about related health professions such as audiology, occupational therapy, physical therapy, and others. These students may seek a career path that is an alternative to a career path in medicine.

Au.D. programs engage in a rigid admissions process that involves submission of materials such as personal statement, graduate record examination scores, official undergraduate transcripts, personal interview, and letters of recommendation. Many programs are highly competitive, with average class sizes of 8 to 12 students. Numbers are kept small, in view of one-on-one mentorship with clinical practicum supervisors (preceptors) and research mentors. Most Au.D. programs are 4 years in length, although some may require students without a background in SHS to take prerequisite courses that could lengthen the program. Conversely, there are 3-year programs in existence and there are also consortium models, whereby several universities in one state may combine resources toward implementation of a program.

Early in their curricula, most programs incorporate scientific foundational courses such as anatomy and physiology, neuroscience, psychoacoustics, hearing and vestibular disorders, and others. Courses reflecting scientific underpinnings are complemented by clinically oriented courses, such as clinical audiology, a hearing device sequence, an electrophysiology sequence, vestibular assessment, aural rehabilitation, hearing conservation, and others. Laboratory-based, hands-on experiences are critical components of such courses, so that the student may apply concepts learned in the classroom and also "bridge" between the classroom and the clinical settings. Statistics and research methods courses are also crucial, so that students may learn consumerism of the literature and skills necessary to study the evidence and apply those principles to daily practice.

A very important component of an Au.D. curriculum is the clinical practicum component, whereby students actually see patients under supervision so that they may apply knowledge learned and skills gained in real-life settings. Au.D. programs vary with regard to when students begin experiencing their clinical placements, with the fourth year (or final year, in the event of a 3-year program) typically considered the full-time clinical externship year. Practicum sites are varied, just as job settings of an audiologist are varied. Audiologists may complete practicum or work in such settings as clinics, hospitals, universities, research laboratories, manufacturing, private practices, not-for-profit organizations, school districts, schools for children who are deaf or hard-of-hearing, and countless other types of facilities. Practicum sites affiliated with an Au.D. program may vary in scope and number, depending upon factors such as the university's geographic location and whether the program is located in a rural versus urban area. Students often obtain clinical practicum experience within the program-housed clinics prior to being placed off-campus or at a site in another city. Appropriate supervision is crucial and is provided in graduated steps, as the student gains more experience and becomes more independent. It is important to ensure quality of sites and supervisors (preceptors) and to coordinate clinical practicum experiences with coursework that the student has completed.

The fourth year externship characteristics also may vary among programs, although many students embark upon the externship after completing coursework, earlier practicum rotations, and any research project that may be required. An externship search and application process is initiated during the fall of the third year of study (sooner if there is a 3-year program), followed by interviewing and making/accepting of offers. The timeline for this process across the country and across sites is highly variable, although AAA has published a recommended timeline for programs, students, sites, and supervisors (preceptors) to follow. Some externs may prefer to stay in the city that houses their program, whereas others may choose to extern at a varied array of sites across the country. The spirit of the externship is toward a depth and breadth of clinical experiences. Just as audiologists may specialize, externs may choose to begin making inroads toward specialization via the externship and example areas may include pediatrics, hearing aids, cochlear implants, adult settings (such as with the veterans administration), and others. Employment options are plentiful, once the student graduates upon completion of the externship and fulfillment of all other graduation requirements. Some students are offered employment, following externing at a particular site. The mentored externship search serves as an admirable "trial run" for the eventual job search. In addition to the variable timeline inherent within the search process, other challenges may include variability in stipend awarded to the student; some sites are able to pay while other sites do not pay. The extern is still a student, as opposed to an employee, and unable to bill for services or collect revenue.

● What Is Accreditation and Why Is It Important?

Most professions are in a position to seek accreditation for their educational programs. Benefits are to protect consumers, ensure programs are meeting specified standards, promote standardization among programs, and strive toward the highest quality of education for students. The Council of Academic Accreditation (CAA) is a body affiliated with ASHA that accredits programs in audiology and also in speech-language pathology. Standards are developed by a body of experts, are peer-reviewed prior to adoption, and are revised regularly so that they remain current.

The current CAA Accreditation Standards for Audiology may be viewed at http://www.asha.org. A new set of Standards has been approved and will go into effect in August 2017. The CAA Standards comprise six major components, with the first requiring information about **administrative structure and governance**. This area requires the program to document such important areas as mission statement, strategic plan, nondiscriminatory policies, program director qualifications, and others. The second section, focusing on **faculty**, specifies such important areas as faculty qualifications, student-faculty ratios, whether faculty members are remaining current, and whether there is a diverse faculty. All standard sections require supporting examples and documentation, such as copies of handbooks, policies, faculty curriculum vitae, curricula and others. The third section requires a program to outline its **curriculum**, ensuring that there is a depth and breadth of experiences that thoroughly cover the scope of practice. Required course content areas are specified, as are areas of skills and knowledge that the student must demonstrate, through integration of didactic coursework with clinical practicum experiences. There are requirements for the scientific underpinnings of clinical practice, as well as the research base such that graduates are skilled at critically analyzing the literature and applying concepts to daily practice. The fourth area targets the **student body**, ensuring that admissions processes are rigorous, that the recruited student body is diverse, that students with alternate learning styles receive proper accommodations, and that proper mechanisms are in place for student advising and mentoring. The fifth area requires a **program** to have assessment tools in place relative to all facets of education. For example, the program may describe formative and summative assessment methods related to such areas as course evaluations, practicum supervisor evaluations of student practicum performance, alumni and employer surveys, and faculty surveys related to major program areas. The sixth and final area relates to **resources**, ensuring financial support, that facilities are conducive to learning, that there is appropriate support staff, and that the program is positioned to flourish and develop further.

The CAA requires a program to submit an accreditation or reaccreditation report, according to a chosen cycle that is typically 5 to 8 years in length. A site visit team is formed that conducts an in-person site visit of the program, typically lasting 2 to 3 days. An annual report is submitted by the program during years when reaccreditation does not take place, with continual oversight by the accrediting body.

The Accreditation Commission for Audiology Education (ACAE) is a second accrediting body that is in existence, having developed approximately 12 years ago. It was developed of, by, and for the profession of audiology and may be accessed at http://www.acaeaccred.org. This organization is affiliated with AAA. There are currently five major areas of Standards, including a general category as the first, whereby programs must describe **governance and policies** that are in place. The second area involves **administrative structure**, whereby programs state goals and how they accomplish goals or outcomes in a measurable way. Programs describe finances and facilities, resources, and recruitment/retention of a high-quality and diverse student body. The third area relates to **planning and evaluation**, where programs must perform self-study and planning, along with assessment that serves to improve various aspects of the program. The fourth area specifies actual **curricular standards**, requiring that students learn via multiple modes of instruction. **Specific knowledge and competency** areas are divided into four subcategories that include **foundational**, **diagnosis and management**, **communication**, and **professional responsibility/values**. This section helps determine if programs are meeting standard requirements for optimal clinical environments, the externship experiences, and projects to foster development of the research foundation. The fifth section relates to **faculty** and ensuring quality, numbers, experiences, and expertise. ACAE Standards have also recently been revised via an expert panel and a peer-review process; they are currently undergoing the adoption process. In a fashion similar to the CAA protocols, ACAE-accredited programs enter data yearly into a web-based platform, undergoing initial accreditation and reaccreditation via self-study, virtual site visit, and face-to-face site visit.

● What Is Certification and What Does It Involve?

It may be common to confuse accreditation with certification. Accreditation, described in a previous section, ensures that **academic programs** are meeting certain standards for high quality education of its students. Certification ensures that the **practitioner** is meeting certain standards, for delivery of high-quality care to patients. ASHA's standards for earning of its CCC may be noted at http://www.asha.org. These standards focus on the following areas: degree received by the applicant, educational program, program of study, knowledge and skills outcomes, assessment, and maintenance of certification. Seeking of certification may be facilitated for a graduate of a CAA-accredited program. To acquire certification, the applicant must also pay a (yearly) fee, pass the national Praxis examination, and abide by the professional organization's code of ethics. Maintenance of certification involves submission of documentation of regular continuing education activities, in the spirit of lifelong learning and remaining current in the field.

The ABA, affiliated with AAA, also offers certification in various specialty areas to its members. Current areas of specialty are pediatric audiology and cochlear implants, with plans underway for certification in precepting/supervising of students. Information is available through http://www.boardofaudiology.org. Applicants must have undergone at least 2,000 hours of mentored professional practice, must pay a fee, and must demonstrate continuous learning. ABA-certified audiologists must recertify every 3 years.

● What Is Licensure?

Each of the 50 states in the United States holds its own state licensing board, with individualized criteria for licensure. An audiologist must be licensed to professionally practice, as a protection of the consumer and testament toward appropriate credentials and competence. Some states offer temporary licensure prior to permanent licensure, for example, for fourth-year externs who may be in final stages of fulfilling degree requirements. With an initial application, many states require payment of a fee and documentation that degree requirements have been met. The applicant may also be required to answer a series of questions, for example, related to past licensure expirations/revocations or any past arrests. Each licensing board carries a mechanism for issuance of complaints, as well as a protocol for licensure renewal on a regularly-scheduled cycle. Such renewal will likely involve payment of a fee, as well as evidence of continuing education credits completed during that particular cycle.

● Why Is Research Important and How Is It Integrated into Au.D. Programs?

The term "evidence-based practice" (EBP) has become a crucial one in medicine, audiology, speech-language pathology, and other professions. Throughout educational programs, students are taught the importance of a strong scientific foundation toward a clinical practice. For example, in audiology the students must know underpinnings such as those relevant to anatomy, physiology, acoustics, and psychoacoustics. They must develop skills of curiosity and inquiry, to perpetuate the scientific and research bases upon which a clinical profession was built. Au.D. students must learn how to critically analyze the literature that appears in peer-reviewed journals. These consumerism of the literature skills promote critical thinking and clinical decision making, enhancing skills of state-of-the-art levels of practice that are sound and based on current evidence. Students also learn theory upon which clinical practice is based, as opposed to merely practicing "cookbook" methodologies.

With the advent of the Au.D. degree within the profession came a dichotomy between that clinically oriented degree and the Doctor of Philosophy (Ph.D.) degree that may be in audiology or the speech and hearing sciences. The latter degree has traditionally been more of a research-oriented degree, and degree recipients have generally been employed in academically-oriented institutions. There is a great deal of overlap between the two degrees in real practice, with recipients of both found in private practice, clinical work, academia, and other settings. Au.D. programs vary with respect to their philosophies related to integration of research within a clinically oriented degree. This author is a strong supporter of maintaining the research base for several reasons, one of which relates to EBP previously described. If a graduate functions strictly as a clinician, the EBP factor is still crucial. There is a shortage of Ph.D. level audiologists. The second reason for exposure to research is to help contribute to the knowledge base of the profession by either educating Au.D. level audiologists to feel comfortable with research skills or to attract them to further education and potential research careers.

Au.D. students may be exposed to research and researchers via numerous avenues. Most curricula include a statistics course and/or a research methodology course. If research is conducted at the home university, students are exposed to research and researchers through jobs as laboratory assistants, coursework, research seminars, local and national meetings, and class projects. Instructors may require assignments whereby the student critiques and discusses peer-reviewed journal articles. This assignment may be complemented by assignment of a research presentation or paper. Within our profession, there is a paucity of professionals who are eligible to serve as members of journal editorial boards and as peer reviewers of submitted manuscripts. Students should be instructed in the spirit of lifelong learning, leadership, and the need for service to the profession. Serving as an editorial board member and/or reviewer is one way to give of one's time and talents. Graduates may also feel an obligation or desire to give back to one's profession via conducting research, sharing of knowledge, presentation at national meetings, mentoring of his/her own students, and/or publication in peer-reviewed (or non-peer-reviewed) journals.

The Au.D. program at Washington University has established a unique Capstone research project model that students complete during the third year of study. Support mechanisms are incorporated during earlier years, such as the statistics and research methods courses, opportunities to familiarize with potential mentors and projects, and human rights protection office training. The proposal is due at the beginning of the third year of study, signed by student, advisor, and second advisor. After approval by the Program Director and Director of Audiology Studies, the student may begin working on the project in earnest. In addition to exposing students to the research process, one goal is toward independent work. Acceptable projects may include a traditional research project via the scientific method, meta-analysis, development of clinical protocol or assessment tool, or development/revision of best practice document. A simple literature review or case study will not suffice. Experiences throughout the year are broad, including gaining skills in scientific writing, literature review, participant recruitment, data collection, sample/effect size calculations, data analysis, development of discussion points, and drawing of conclusions. A Capstone Guidebook, revised on a yearly basis, has been developed by the program, to outline procedures for students and mentors. Students present their research at the program's annual Student Research Colloquium, which takes place at the end of each academic year. Capstone papers are published in Washington University's Becker Library Digital Repository; many are of such high quality that they are accepted for presentation at local and national meetings and/or submitted for publication in peer-reviewed journals.

Optional research experiences for students are also plentiful within the program. Students often become involved in investigators' research laboratories soon after enrollment and this may take place throughout the entire 4 years of study. Although the externship is a clinically oriented experience, many sites offer research experiences so that students may complement their clinical practicum experiences. There are summer research traineeships for which students may apply, supported by the National Institutes of Health, National Institute for Deafness and Other Communication Disorders, and various national organizations. Some grant funding may also offer a pull-out year of research, embedded within the 4 years of Au.D. study, allowing the possibility of earning an additional degree. Rich integration of research into a rigorous, clinically oriented curriculum helps to proliferate creation of new knowledge and to embrace development of evidence-based practitioners. Many graduates seek employment where they balance clinical with research work, whereas others may plan to further their education via a more research-oriented Ph.D. degree.

● Are Au.D. Students Involved in Interprofessional Education?

It is well known that a team approach in patient assessment and management is optimal, such that clinicians may manage the "whole patient" and his/her family. Interprofessional education (IPE) knowledge and skills are mandated in accreditation standards of many other health-related professions. Such knowledge and skills are becoming mandated within the profession of audiology, as indicated by new accreditation standards that are in process, and it is important that such experiences be incorporated into educational programs. Audiologists must learn to work effectively with professionals in medicine, nursing, pharmacy, occupational therapy, physical therapy, social work, speech-language pathology, deaf education, and myriad others. One basic, guiding principle of IPE is that learners must engage in enriched opportunities to learn with and from other professions' learners.

Washington University School of Medicine in St. Louis has just proudly launched its new Center for Interprofessional Practice and Education (CIPE), in collaboration with the Goldfarb School of Nursing and the St. Louis College of Pharmacy. CIPE's Curriculum Committee is in the process of reviewing and integrating all professional accreditation standards and curricula and is also developing activities and learning modules for facilitation of IPE. All first-year students are required to attend three sessions at the current time, with goals of learning more about each of the other professions. Teams are developed for the learning opportunities, as students learn roles and responsibilities of each profession. Team-building activities are implemented that foster enhanced teamwork and open communication. Case studies related to actual patients are beneficial, so that each learner understands his/her role and also the important role of others. While there are many models for implementing IPE, execution of the following domains are important, including at Washington University. Domains are modeled after core competencies for interprofessional collaborative practice (2011).[1] The area of **values and ethics** is important, so that students learn to value and respect cultural diversity, inclusion, development of trust on the part of the patient and among team members, and cooperative work. Development of knowledge related to **roles and responsibilities** of self and team members is also critical. All professionals must recognize limitations, appropriate referral mechanisms, provision of complementary services, high standards of care (individually and as a team), effective communication, and growing interdependence upon other team members. Exercising of exemplary **interprofessional communication skills** is a critical component, including consideration of patients and families as valued team members. Professionals must learn to listen to patients well and to implement patient-centered and community-focused assessment and treatment. Finally, **teams and teamwork** are necessary for effective integration of all professions' contributions. Team members develop together toward effective leadership, constructive ways to disagree, efficient strategies for strengthening teamwork, and team practice that are based on the most current evidence.

It is beneficial when an audiology program is housed within a vibrant medical school, where students have vast opportunities to take part in a wide array of excellent learning opportunities with world-recognized professionals. Within the Au.D. program at Washington University and specifically related to collaboration with otolaryngology, the students have opportunities for a boundless array of research topics and endeavors, shadowing of physicians as they treat patients, observation of surgery, hands-on dissections within temporal bone banks, attendance at audiology and ENT grand rounds, exposure to regular brown-bag research seminars, and countless additional ones. Conversely, resident and attending physicians have much to learn from audiologists with respect to assessment and its interpretation, as well as a multitude of treatment strategies from newborn through geriatric patients.

As audiologists work closely with otolaryngologists, such teamwork and mutual respect develop. The audiologist holds a doctoral degree, accompanied by rigorous coursework and extensive clinical practicum experience. The audiologist is not viewed as a technician who merely "turns dials," as the profession encompasses so much more. Rather, the audiologist works side-by-side in clinical decision making, counseling, imparting recommendations, follow-up care, and much more.

What Are Other "Hot Topics" in Au.D. Education?

The Au.D. degree has now been offered for over 20 years, and it has evolved from primarily a distance-learning "retooling" for those holding master's degrees to extensive, typically 4-year residency programs that have been described. As with any profession, there is continual self-assessment related to areas that are working well versus those that could be modified. Also as with any profession, audiologists are adapting to health care changes and reimbursement rate challenges. No one knows what the future has in store, but development of critical thinking skills help to effectively navigate challenges. It is not enough to learn to become highly competent with each patient who makes his/her way into one's clinic. Rather, one must also exercise leadership, advocacy for one's profession and patients, exceptional communication and professional writing skills, sharing of knowledge, visibility, presentation skills, and a sense of "giving back" to one's profession. Audiologists' scope of practice is ever evolving and expanding, while advancements in technology are exploding. Areas of specialization are continually evolving, with audiologists gaining more autonomy with respect to services provided. Professionals must remain current, including with respect to lifelong learning and keeping up with current evidence.

It has become increasingly necessary for Au.D. students to take more business-related courses and for audiologists to accrue business-related skills. Development of private practices are becoming more common, along with prior-mentioned evolution toward greater autonomy. Audiologists are often the entry point into hearing health care for a patient who is deaf or hard-of-hearing. In addition to knowledge surrounding billing and reimbursement, clinicians must be well-versed in accounting, analysis of profit/loss, marketing of services, recruitment of patients, supervision of office personnel, and overall managing of a practice. These skills are highly important when employed in other settings, as well. The profession has been rated by various surveys as being highly fulfilling and desirable. There is also a need for audiologists, especially as medical care helps to promote infant survival rate and as our population of older citizens increases.

What Does the Future Hold for Au.D. Education, as the Foundation for the Profession?

As with any relatively new profession and any recently implemented degree, there must be ongoing assessment related to areas that must be improved. Governing bodies and leadership must also exercise dynamic, as opposed to static, management to keep up with a transitioning climate and expanding scope of practice. Although it is admirable that founding fathers of the Au.D. degree demonstrated the vision and building blocks for implementation, there are important areas to address in the future. Previously described development of leadership and critical thinking in current students and future leaders may be key principles in ensuring successful proliferation of the profession. Certainly, a rigorous and thorough curriculum within our educational programs is a critical foundation for development of such future leaders.

One pressing concern is that the students accrue significant debt load, upon graduation from a 4-year doctoral program. Two years of graduate debt load has transitioned to 4 years of graduate debt load, along with the profession's transition from entry-level master's to doctoral degree. Graduates' debt load may vary, depending upon such factors as compounding undergraduate debt load, tuition rates at state-supported versus private universities, and sources of funding throughout the graduate educational program. Although educational requirements to become an audiologist have increased, along with debt load, salaries have not necessarily done so. Although audiologists must strive toward increasing salaries that are commensurate with service and debt load, this becomes challenging in a health care climate of diminishing reimbursement rates.

Audiology has traditionally been housed, at least on an undergraduate educational level, along with its "sister" profession of speech-language pathology. Although these two professions have similar foundations, there has also been divergence with one major area being a master's degree versus a doctoral degree as entry level into the profession. There is great variability in administrative structure in which Au.D. programs are housed, including within medical schools, departments of education, Colleges of Arts and Sciences, departments of public or allied health, and many others. Although audiologists are employed in schools and other settings, there appears to be a migration toward a more medically-oriented model, as we see with medicine, occupational therapy, pharmacy, physical therapy, and other health-related professions. It is possible that medical models of these other professions could serve as a base for transition within audiology. That is, the externship could potentially be streamlined and discussion could take place related to some type of residency model that occurs post-graduation. This would be for the purpose of refinement of skills and/or specialization.

Three-year programs have developed, as discussed, and student debt load must be considered. Currently, there is an inequity between 3- and 4-year programs that will become standardized in the future, along with standardization in other important areas. Founding fathers envisioned a smaller number of Au.D. programs when the profession transitioned toward a doctoral degree for entry. This was accompanied by a greater student enrollment per program. Factors that limit enrollment must be overcome, such as securing mentors for Capstone research projects and sufficient clinical practicum experiences for all. One-on-one clinical practicum experiences with patients and supervisors will be enhanced via technological advances such as telehealth, experiences in actor–patient laboratories, and simulations of real-life patient experiences. To facilitate the field's proliferation, it will be helpful to consider unification with respect to educational program accrediting bodies and certification bodies of individual practitioners. There appears to be a need for a greater number of audiologists accompanying enhancement of audiology service provision, particularly as the infant mortality rate diminishes and as health care advances lead to life longevity with the elderly. Along with greater enrollments within educational programs will possibly come an increased role of the audiology assistant. These individuals may be trained to provide less-sophisticated tasks, such as electroacoustic analysis of hearing devices, basic hearing aid repairs, screening, perhaps some basic components of the behavioral/electrophysiologic battery, and others. The primary audiologist would provide a supervisory role and a major responsibility would be toward performance of more sophisticated measures, interpretation of results, and overall management of the whole patient. Interprofessional education will continue to flourish, as a fine balance is attained of finding common threads toward working together versus avoidance of service duplication. Quality control will be ensured, with emphasis upon rigorous education, focus upon best practice, and highest quality of service provision that is based on latest of evidence in the literature. As audiologists experience optimum education that includes scientific foundation, clinical skills and knowledge, and extensive practicum experiences, they are well poised to work closely with otolaryngologists and other professionals. All collectively exercise optimal clinical decision making, with the common goal of providing the highest quality of hearing health care to patients across the lifespan and their families.

Reference

1. Interprofessional Education Collaborative Expert Panel. Core compe-
    tencies for interprofessional collaborative practice: report of an expert
    panel. Washington, DC: Interprofessional Education Collaborative; 2011

Index

Page number in *italics* refer to illustrations; those in **bold** refer to tables